Female Sex Anomalies

Female Sex Anomalies

Cary M. Dougherty, M.D.

Clinical Professor, Department of Obstetrics and Gynecology,
Louisiana State University School of Medicine; Senior Visiting Surgeon,
Charity Hospital of Louisiana at New Orleans, Active Medical Staff,
Woman's Hospital; Active Medical Staff, Earl K. Long Hospital, Baton Rouge

Rowena Spencer, M.D.

Clinical Associate Professor of Surgery (Pediatric Surgery),
Tulane University School of Medicine, New Orleans; Senior Visiting Surgeon,
Charity Hospital of Louisiana at New Orleans; Senior, Active Staff,
Touro Infirmary, New Orleans

WITH 4 CONTRIBUTORS

WITH 141 ILLUSTRATIONS

Medical Department
HARPER & ROW, PUBLISHERS
Hagerstown, Maryland
New York, Evanston, San Francisco, and London

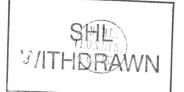

First Edition

Standard Book Number: 06-140694-5

Library of Congress Catalog Card Number: 71-187045

Contents

v

Contributors

CARY M. DOUGHERTY, M.D.

Clinical Professor, Department of Obstetrics and Gynecology, Louisiana State University School of Medicine; Senior Visiting Surgeon, Charity Hospital of Louisiana at New Orleans; Active Medical Staff, Woman's Hospital; Active Medical Staff, Earl K. Long Hospital, Baton Rouge

ADOLPH H. SELLMANN, M.D.

Associate Professor, Department of Obstetrics and Gynecology, Louisiana State University School of Medicine, New Orleans; Project Director, Child Development Study, Charity Hospital of Louisiana at New Orleans

ROWENA SPENCER, M.D.

Clinical Associate Professor of Surgery (Pediatric Surgery), Tulane University School of Medicine, New Orleans; Senior Visiting Surgeon, Charity Hospital of Louisiana at New Orleans; Senior, Active Staff, Touro Infirmary, New Orleans

JOHN C. WEED, M.D.

Clinical Professor of Obstetrics and Gynecology, Tulane University School of Medicine; Head, Department of Obstetrics and Gynecology, Ochsner Foundation Hospital, New Orleans

Preface

For lack of proper understanding, individuals having anomalous sex organs are regarded as freaks, persons who cannot fit in. Our current social order can comprehend no sexual subdivisions other than "male" and "female"—either one or the other. It is not to deprecate common medical knowledge of the subject to say that many persons do not understand the difference between the intersex and the homosex, between anomalous sexual anatomy and anomalous sexual behavior. These persons seem to expect the hermaphroditic newborn to grow up to be a sexual deviate or pervert. Other equally erroneous ideas may be found among nonmedical and medical persons regarding those individuals born without a vagina, those who have breasts when they shouldn't, those without the usual accessory sex characteristics, or those without normal sex organs of one type or the other. With this general background of misinformation, the average person finds it difficult to understand that there are many types and degrees of hermaphroditism in the human being and that possession of anatomically in-between or malformed sex organs does not necessarily predetermine an abnormal life.

To clarify the facts concerning anatomic abnormalities of the reproductive organs, we thought it appropriate to list the different conditions by major organ affected. This decision is sometimes counter to the current trend of classification by chromosomal pattern, but is more useful to the physician who must see and examine the patient with the anomaly.

An important part of the understanding of anomalous development is the knowledge of the events of normal development—embryology. To stress the importance of knowing normal embryology of the genital organs, we have compiled a detailed account of this fascinating event in the first chapter and at the beginning of the chapter on congenital adrenal cortical hyperplasia. A short review of the embryology of the respective sex organs precedes each chapter. Let no one underestimate the importance of embryology in the study of developmental defects in the human female.

ix

There is a natural separation of cases into three categories according to age at which the signs of abnormality are first noted, although this age is being steadily pushed back to unity by better understanding and diagnosis. In the *intrauterine period* the anomaly may be of such great magnitude that spontaneous termination of the pregnancy takes place. Anatomic studies of abortuses, including the ovum, embryo, and fetus, reveal interesting facts concerning pathologic development of the sex organs. Congenital anomalies likely to be discovered in the *neonatal period* are those of the external genitalia, anus, sacrum, pubis, and urinary apparatus, i.e., defects of the hind end of the body. When the female child reaches the period of *sexual maturity*, the signs of anomaly are a failure in the functioning of the three major acts associated with sexual maturity: menstruation, coitus, and pregnancy.

In those instances where something can be done to correct nature's mistake the diagnostic work-up must be early and thorough. A plan of treatment should be laid out which not only stipulates the proper surgical and hormonal measures to be carried out, but also formulates a schedule by which the correct procedure is done at the correct time.

Case histories used in the monograph came from the files of Charity Hospital at New Orleans, from records of consultations of the authors, and from the records of the careful dissections of the fetuses collected by Dr. Rowena Spencer. Where possible the patients were contacted and brought in for further examining and testing. Our work, therefore, is based mainly on our own experiences. We make no claim of having catalogued all the many rare and unusual varieties of intersex and of anomalous conditions of the reproductive system in the human female.

The discovery of the sex chromatin mass in the interphase nucleus and the perfection of techniques for chromosome counting have increased our knowledge of chromosomal aberrations and their role in sex anomalies. So important is this phase of diagnostic study that we believe the medical practitioner should not even attempt management of the patient with genital defects unless he has access to laboratory facilities for accurate and repeated chromosomal typing.

The complicated surgical procedures used in some of these cases should be learned of by reading about them, but skill required to accomplish them must necessarily be acquired by precept.

C. M. D.

Acknowledgments

To Nadalyn Cotten goes credit for most of the literary effort and a major part of scientific skill required in preparing this monograph. The authors feel that her contributions were among the essentials, without which our job could not have been done. Further superlatives are but inadequate to describe her talents in turning out the finished product.

Members of the medical staff of Charity Hospital and the Louisiana State University School of Medicine who have a special interest in endocrinology have been most helpful in allowing us to cite their case records. Among these are Drs. William Blackard, Douglass Gordon, and Robert Weilbaecher. Members of the Department of Pediatrics—who seem to be preempting the field by their earlier and earlier recognition of the sexually anomalous newborn—have been especially cooperative in supplying information in these cases. Particular acknowledgments are due Drs. Curtis Johnson and Theodore Thurmond and the director of the department, Dr. Richard Fowler.

My colleagues in Baton Rouge have been both interested and helpful in informing us of anomalous developments in their patients and in allowing us to carry out investigations of these individuals. Mrs. Rita Bondio of the Medical Records Department of Charity Hospital was particularly helpful in locating patients' charts. Dr. Spencer's collection of fetuses was made possible by a grant from the Schlieder Foundation. And last, the members of the Department of Obstetrics-Gynecology, and the director, Abe Mickal, have contributed greatly in finding and managing the patients in whom we have special medical interest and concern.

Our sincere thanks go to all these fine persons.

Female Sex Anomalies

Chapter One

Genesis of the Female Reproductive System

Cary M. Dougherty and A. H. Sellmann

Construction of the complete female reproductive system is contracted for as soon as an X-chromosome-bearing spermatozoon meets and fertilizes the ovum. The first morphologic signs of the development of this repository for and transmitter of eternal germ plasm do not, however, show up for 3 weeks. From that point on there is steady activity in its construction until, in the 180-mm fetus, the entire tract is completed in an immature nonfunctional—but receptive to maturing and functioning—form.

The embryonic parts composing the genital system are gonad, wolffian (mesonephric) duct, müllerian (paranephric) duct, urogenital sinus, and external genitals (genital tubercle).

SEX DETERMINATION AND SEX DIFFERENTIATION

In higher animals and in humans maleness and femaleness are predetermined genetically, i.e., by mechanisms involving chromosomes. Since chromosomal determination of sex differentiation is a relatively new evolutionary mechanism, the human embryo in recapitulating phylogeny goes through a long period of development in which it is indifferent sexually, or in a sense bisexual (except for carrying one or the other of the sex-determining chromosomes). Germ cells have been identified in the very early human embryo (1+ mm), long before the gonadal anlage appears. From the original site they migrate to the gonad (5–8 mm), and only then are they induced to develop as ovogonia or spermatogonia. As far as can be determined at the present, there is no difference (except chromosomal content) between primitive germ cells destined to form ovogonia and those which will form spermatogonia. Gonocytes (primi-

TABLE 1-1

TIME TABLE OF DEVELOPMENT OF THE FEMALE GENITAL TRACT

Size (mm)	(Age weeks) *	
.08	7.5 days	Bilaminar disc embryo
.21	13 days	Yolk sac forming, hindgut, foregut
.36	20 days	Allantois formed
1.5	2+	Gonocytes are located in yolk sac entoderm
		Urogenital ridge begins to form
2	3	Wolffian duct appears as coalescence of pronephric ducts
		Allantois well formed, joins hindgut at cloaca
		Cloacal membrane forms as cloaca contacts hind end ectoderm
4	4	Wolffian ducts open into urogenital sinus (cloaca)
5		Primordium of gonad appears
6	4+	Primordial germ cells in mesenchyme
7	1 mo+	Indifferent gonad developing
	5	Wolffian ducts open to urogenital sinus
		Ureteric buds
		External genital tubercle forming
8		Sex cords budding from celomic epithelium
		Anlage of adrenal cortex forms
		Urorectal septum starts partition of cloaca
10		Free ends of sex cords form rete testis
11	5.5	Müllerian funnel and duct begin to form
		Primary bifurcation of ureteric bud
		Sex difference in external genitalia: urethral groove shorter in female
		Urethral folds develop lateral to central groove
15	5¾	Differentiation of gonad into testis in male
		Ureter opens separately from Wolffian duct into urogenital sinus
16	6	Cloaca subdividing. Urorectal septum completed
		Phallus forming from genital tubercle
18		Secondary bifurcation of ureteric bud
		Urethral membrane (and cloacal membrane) perforate
20	7	Gonad recognizable as ovary; cortex forming
		Labioscrotal folds developed (lateral genital swellings)
23	8	

TABLE 1-1 (Continued)

TIME TABLE OF DEVELOPMENT OF THE FEMALE GENITAL TRACT

Size (mm)	(Age weeks) *	
25		Coronary sulcus of phallus appears
		Female phallus shows caudal curvature
30		Interstitial cells recognizable
32	9	Müllerian ducts reach urogenital sinus
		Müllerian tubercle formed
42		Lower müllerian ducts fused
45	10	Wolffian ducts begin to regress in female
		Coronary sulcus of phallus forms groove easily recognized
50		Posterior commissure formed
		Great increase of Leydig cells from mesenchyme
		Prostatic buds first appear in male
56	11	Sex differences in external genitals first noticeable
		Uterovaginal canal formed, fusion of müllerian ducts with sinovaginal bulbs
65		Wolffian ducts begin to disappear
		Longitudinal folds in urogenital sinus
		Sinovaginal bulbs formed, obliterate müllerian tubercle
70	12	Beginning solidification of uterovaginal canal by "proliferation of both müllerian and sinovaginal" epithelium
94		Sinus upgrowth along vaginal plate
100	16	Wolffian ducts have disappeared by this stage
		External genitalia of male fully formed
125		Fetal ovarian stroma differentiates
150		Primordial follicles in central part of ovary
		Vagina canalizes from urogenital sinus forward
		Maximum development of Leydig cells
175	20	Beginning shrinking and degeneration of Leydig cells
180		Vagina fully canalized; glycogenated epithelium
187		Seminiferous tubules coiled; lumina
200	24	
240	7 mo (early)	Testes descend into scrotum
250	28	During cortical differentiation, medullary cords crowded centrally; some medullary tubules provided with germ cells persist in hilum
286	32	Reduction in Leydig cells (male)
		Disappearance of medullary cords in ovary (female)

* Except as otherwise noted.

tive germ cells) cannot self-differentiate, but are probably dependent upon a special influence of the gonadal primordia for this purpose. Those in the medulla of one type of gonad form spermatogonia, while those in the cortex of the other type of gonad form ovogonia.[19]

The developing gonad goes through a long period in which testis and ovary are indistinguishable by morphologic criteria. At a critical time (14- to 20-mm stage by morphologic indicators) chromosomal influences, sex inductors,[21] steroid hormones, or a combination of these act upon the indifferent gonad to produce medullary predominance (maleness) or cortical predominance (femaleness).

The continued development of male and female reproductive apparatuses proceeds in a predictable and explainable fashion (Table 1-1). Successive steps are built on the immediately antecedent ones, like dominoes placed on dominoes. In the indifferent stage two sets of sex ducts are laid out: wolffian for male use and müllerian for female purposes. The lower urogenital tract and the urogenital sinus internally, as well as the genital tubercle externally, are of the same form in the early male and female fetuses. Specific differentiation takes place in one set of genital ducts probably as a result of its being stimulated preferentially by the gonad, while the other set undergoes atrophy due to inhibitory substance from the same source.[19] Under male gonadal influence the urogenital sinus produces urethra, prostate, and urethral glands, while female gonads condition urethra, periurethral glands, vagina, and vaginal vestibule.

Thus, the development of the genital system in the long indifferent stage allows the occasion for operation of abnormal influences, both chromosomal and external, which produce all intermediate shades of abnormality of the system, depending upon the exact time at which they are operational.

The relation between the crown-rump length (CRL) of the fetus and its age is shown in Table 1-2.

TABLE 1-2
RELATION BETWEEN SIZE AND AGE OF FETUS

Crown-rump length (mm)	Age	
	Weeks	Months (lunar)
0 – 2.5	4	1
2.6– 25	8	2
26 – 68	12	3
69 –121	16	4
122 –167	20	5
168 –210	24	6
211 –245	28	7
246 –284	32	8
285 –316	36	9
317 –336	40	10

Data from Mall, F. P., and Meyer, A. W.: Studies on abortuses: A survey of pathologic ova in the Carnegie embryological collection. **Contrib Embryol 12:**199, 1921.

GONADS (5–20 mm)

The beginning of the genital system may be seen in the appearance of the urogenital ridges, one on either side of the dorsal mesentery of the gut, very early in embryonic life (Fig. 1-1). The beginning of the gonad is evident when in the 5-mm embryo there is thickening of the celomic epithelial covering of the underside of the mesenchymal bulges and a condensation of the mesenchyme proper just deep to the covering. The wolffian duct is already formed by coalition of the very early appearing pronephric tubules, and the mesonephros is starting to form its glomeruli when the first features of the gonad are evident. The paired ridges are appropriately designated the *urogenital ridges.*

Origins of the Gonad

The medial longitudinal portion of *mesenchyme* of the urogenital ridge forms gonadal stroma. Extending from one end of the celom to the other, this mesenchymal mass is composed of loosely arranged long spindle cells, oriented in a random fashion. Immediately beneath the surface epithelium, the mesenchyme is more condensed, with possibly vertically set cells predominating.[6] Growth of the mesenchymal mass is indicated by presence of many cells in mitosis. In the gonad differentiated as ovary the mesenchyme will form the ovarian cortical stroma and at least the theca layers of the follicle.

The *celomic epithelium* (mesothelium, future peritoneum) covering the gonadal ridge plays an important role in development. At first a thin layer of flattened mesodermal cells, it soon grows into a layer of tall columnar cells and then into a multilayered strip. The epithelium, traditionally called germinal, is separated from the mesenchyme by a thin condensation of eosin-stained material, but this film cannot be traced continuously throughout the extent of the gonad and is not regarded as an intact basement membrane. As development proceeds the germinal epithelium sends masses of epithelial cells into the mesenchymal mass, forming in the case of the male the primary sex cords which are the forerunners of the seminiferous tubules.

Comparable sex cords derived from the germinal epithelium in the young differentiating ovary are not nearly so easy to find. Older embryologists described cords in the testis but not in the ovary. Gillman stated that Fischel (1930) believed that cord-like structures in the ovary were derived from the mesenchymal stroma and gave origin to the entire organ (except ova).[6] His concept recognized the possibility of multipotency of the mesenchymal cell, an important premise in postulating origin of

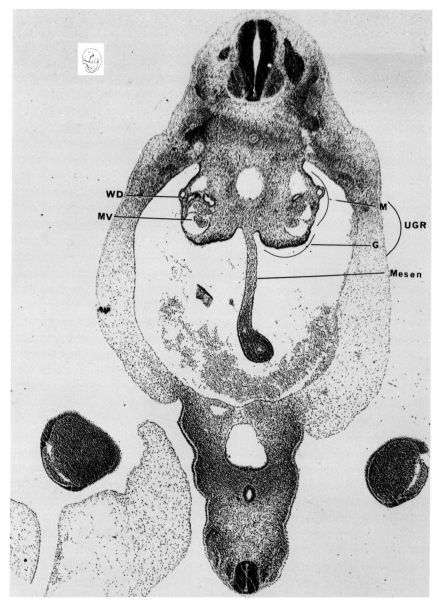

Fig. 1-1. Composition of urogenital ridges. Embryo 6508, 36-3-3; 7.3 mm, 4½ weeks. Bilateral bulges from urogenital ridges (*UGR*) in dorsomedial wall of celomic cavity on either side of mesentery (*Mesen*) of gut. Urogenital ridges (*UGR*) give rise to mesonephros, ovary, and metanephros. Mesonephric (wolffian) vesicles (*MV*) and ducts (*WD*) are completed, and gonadal anlagen (*G*) are evident as masses of mesenchyme covered by thickened celomic epithelium medial to mesonephric apparatus (*M*). 30×. (From Dougherty, C. M. *Surgical Pathology of Gynecologic Disease.* New York, Harper & Row, 1968.)

some types of ovarian tumors, e.g., granulosa—theca cell tumor.[23] Other authors believed that while the germinal epithelium contributes accretions to the gonadal mass it does not actually form cords.[16] The cord-like arrangement results, it is said, from division of the cells of the gonadal blastema into columns by the radially oriented blood vessels of the gonad.

Probably a majority of embryologists consider that the germinal epithelium does contribute a system of primary or medullary cords in the ovary like the sex cords in the testis.[4, 14, 18] In the female these cords are short-lived, for they are soon crowded to the center region by a second proliferation of epithelial cells which forms cortex with cortical or secondary cords. Those in the medulla eventually disappear and are not found in the postnatal ovary. The cortical cords form the granulosa of the ovarian follicle and elicit a reaction of thecal differentiation from the adjacent stromal cells.[6, 19]

The *germ cells* (gonocytes) of the ovary are probably "derived from primordial germ cells, which arise long before the rudiments of the genital folds, and which in embryos of less than 16 somites (2.5 mm, 22 days) are located in the yolk-sac endoderm." [22] Embryologists generally agree that the gonocytes arise in an extragonadal site and reach the gonad by migratory movement. Evidence supporting this view came from morphologic studies of human embryos,[5, 8, 11, 15, 22] as well as from studies of comparative embryology and from experimental embryology.[17] The contribution of Witschi was decisive in establishing the concept of germ cell migration in the human.[22] Oddly enough, a substantial part of his observations resulted from the study of an embryologic specimen contributed by the gynecologic service of Charity Hospital at New Orleans (Carnegie No. 7889). Large clear cells with spherical nuclei containing prominent nucleoli were seen in the yolk sac and in the hindgut in the 3- to 4-mm embryos. These same cells were traced in successively larger embryos in the mesenchyme of the gut, in the mesentery, and more laterally in the mass of the gonadal blastema. In the indifferent gonad these large distinctive cells accumulated in the subepithelial and epithelial regions and eventually became associated with sex cords of the ovary and testis. Witschi was able to trace the paths of these germ cells using histologic appearance alone. McKay *et al.* and Pinkerton *et al.* made essentially the same observations by identifying the germ cells by their strong alkaline phosphatase reaction in tissue sections.

One may fairly safely conclude at this time, then, that gonocytes of the human gonad wander in from another site early in its formation. This site is probably near or in the endoderm of the hindgut and yolk sac, where these specialized cells develop along with the endodermal epithelium. Witschi is of the opinion that the transfer is brought about by the active, ameboid movement of the germ cells guided perhaps by chemotaxis, propelling themselves through the mesenchyme of the dorsal mesentery and thence laterally, reaching the gonadal blastema.

One may now state with all reasonable assurance which structures in the adult organs are derived from each of the three original sources. The germinal epithelium contributes Sertoli cells of the seminiferous tubules, the rete testis, follicular granulosa cells, and the vestigial rete ovarii. The mesenchyme differentiates into interstitial cells of the testis (Leydig cells), interfollicular ovarian cortical stroma, and thecal layers of the follicle. The gonocytes, of course, become spermatogonia and primary ovocytes.

The Indifferent State

From the time the gonadal blastema is first recognizable as a condensation of the mesenchymal cells and a thickening of the celomic epithelium of the genital bulge to the time when it has the morphologic features of ovary (17–20 mm, 5–7 weeks), there are no characteristics (excepting sex chromatin in the nuclei of cells of the ovary) distinguishing testis from ovary, although development proceeds at a rapid pace. Embryologists call this stage of formation the indifferent stage.

Along the underside of the mesonephric eminence the celomic epithelium may be seen to be composed of taller columnar-type cells. At first only a single layer of cells, the epithelium (5 mm, 4 weeks) proliferates until it is made up of several layers of crowded cells. Very active mitotic division is evident. At this early stage one may find the large, pale-stained germ cells in the mesenchyme of the gonadal mass and in the epithelial layer as well. The time-order of appearance of germ cells within mesenchyme and within epithelium has been used as supporting evidence that these cells migrate into the gonad, for they are at first more numerous in the gonadal stroma.

If one does not expect to find discrete, well-formed columns of cells making them up, one could say that at 8 mm, $5\frac{1}{2}$ weeks there are the first visible signs of formation of the primary sex cords of the indifferent or bipotent gonad. The "sex cords" are masses of epithelial cells originating from the surface, pushed inward perhaps by the proliferation of surface cells. At this stage the cord arrangement is indistinct. At once the deeper of the germ cells become associated with the developing cords, and lose some of their distinctive characteristics. The testis may be recognized as early as 14–15 mm, $5\frac{3}{4}$ weeks, by the organization of definite sex cords and by the absence of ovogonia. The ovary is distinctive at about 17–20 mm, 6 weeks, with its large germ cells, the ovogonia, and its less well-differentiated sex cords. From this period onward the development of the male and the female gonads proceeds in diverging paths, medullary elements predominating in the case of testis, cortical components in the case of ovary.

WOLFFIAN DUCT (2–30 mm)

Described by and named after Kaspar Wolff (1733–1794), the mesonephric ducts form the important conduit, the vas deferens, in the male genital system and contribute minor vestiges in the mature female. Beginnings of the duct are found in the 4- to 12-somite embryo (2 mm, 22 days) when the pronephric tubules coalesce to form the pronephric duct. It is located in the lateral portion of the nephrogenic ridge. A simple tube of moderately tall cuboidal cells, the wolffian duct runs lengthwise from cranial to caudal, connecting along the way with the short transverse mesonephric tubules, and reaching the cloacal region at about the 3.5-mm, 4-week stage. Shortly thereafter it opens into the urogenital sinus portion of the cloaca. By the time the embryo has reached 7–8 mm, 4–4½ weeks, the entire mesonephros is well developed and supplied by multiple arteries. There are some 83 pairs of mesonephric tubules and about half that number of glomeruli connected with the wolffian duct (Fig. 1-2).[10]

In the caudal region near the point where the wolffian duct joins the urogenital sinus the duct gives rise to a bud from its dorsal wall (6 mm, 4 weeks). The *ureteric bud* enlarges, divides into secondary and tertiary divisions, ultimately forming ureter and kidney pelvis and collecting tubules of the definitive kidney. Enlarging into the mesenchyme of the metanephrogenic blastema, the ureteric bud elicits a condensation of tissue which differentiates into metanephric cortex: the definitive kidney. By a process of selective growth of the urogenital sinus, the end of the ureteric bud near the sinus leaves the wolffian duct and joins the pars pelvina of the sinus above the junction of the wolffian duct.

MÜLLERIAN DUCTS (11–32 mm)

Long after the gonadal ridge is discernible as a subdivision of the mesonephros and after the wolffian duct has developed in its entirety, the beginnings of the genital ductal system of the female appear. The *müllerian funnel* is first evident in the 11 mm-, 5-week embryo as a groove or depression in the very cranial-most end of the urogenital ridge. The opening of the funnel, eventually forming the ostium and fimbriated end of the fallopian tube, is surrounded by lacy proliferations of the

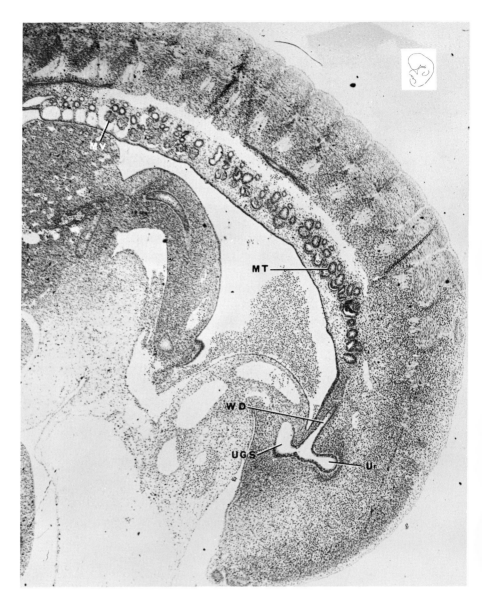

Fig. 1-2. Relations of mesonephros, mesonephric duct, and ureteric bud. Embryo 6504, 12-3-2; 7.5 mm, 4½ weeks. This paramedian sagittal section goes through entire length of the mesonephros, demonstrating its vesicles (*MV*) and tubules (*MT*) and their association with mesonephric duct (*WD*). Duct opens into urogenital sinus (*UGS*) caudally and gives rise to ureteric bud (*Ur*), seen as a dorsally situated bulb in immediate vicinity of sinus. Beginning of metanephros is seen as a condensation of mesenchymal cells about bud. 30×. (From Dougherty, C. M. *Surgical Pathology of Gynecologic Disease*. New York, Harper & Row, 1968.)

celomic epithelium some of which form secondary openings into the funnel. Thus, the ostium is more than a simple opening. As development proceeds the lacework forms the fimbria and the funnel forms a single channel. The caudal end of the funnel extends by growing through the mesenchymal tissues of the ridge just to the outside of the wolffian duct. The backward growth of the müllerian duct is so predictable that its length has been used by embryologists as one of the landmarks of the developmental stage of the embryo. In transverse sections of the mesonephros the wolffian and müllerian ducts may be seen side by side, the müllerian slightly larger and not connected to any lateral tubules.

The müllerian duct in its early phase of formation is essentially a tube of single-layered epithelium, cells of which are cuboidal or columnar. In the cranial end the epithelium is the same as--not a derivative of but the same as—that which covered the mesonephros, it being folded inward in the first formative maneuvers. It is thus a mesodermal epithelium. The remainder of the duct, that part which pushes backward by multiplication of cells at the tip, is composed of epithelium descended from the original celomic lining. Further caudally and further along in its development the simple epithelial tube becomes sheathed in a more closely arranged mass of mesenchymal tissue.

The müllerian duct growing caudally through the mesenchyme follows a course beside the wolffian duct all the way. But while the major part of that course is on the lateral side of the wolffian duct, the müllerian duct makes an S-shaped turn near the pelvic region crossing the wolffian duct ventrally and lying to the medial side as they both come down to the urogenital sinus. In this zone the caudal portions of the paired müllerian ducts are in apposition. The rounded caudal ends, closed by a few layers of müllerian epithelium, come to rest against the epithelium of the dorsal wall of the urogenital sinus, there to await localized phenomena shortly to take place in the urogenital sinus epithelium.

At the place where the two müllerian ducts touch the sinus wall, there is a small indentation of the wall into the lumen of the sinus, a concentration of mesenchyme about the ends of the müllerian ducts, and most conspicuously, proliferation of the sinus epithelium and differentiation into a multilayered, clear-cell type. These three elements combine to form a little mound, the müllerian tubercle, protruding into the lumen of the sinus. A small but important feature of the formation of tissue at this point is the wisp of mesenchyme in the middle at the blunt ends of the two müllerian ducts. Persistence and enlargement of this bit of connective tissue is an element in production of a vaginal septum.

UROGENITAL SINUS (2–50 mm)

In the very early embryo the hindgut ends in a blind pouch, its caudal tip resting against an area of ectoderm near the tail known as the *cloacal plate.* In the region of the hindgut a ventral diverticulum is formed by evagination of the gut. It extends out as part of the body stalk (2–3 mm, 24 days). This structure is the *allantois,* a primitive excretory organ in lower animals. It is destined to take part in the formation of the lower genital tract and the lower urinary tract.

In the beginning the allantois is simply a diverticulum from the gut (allantoenteric diverticulum) sloping back and joining the gut in an over-and-under fashion in the caudal region. Soon, however, the common cloaca is partitioned lengthwise in a frontal plane by a septum, the *urorectal fold.* In the 14- to 16-mm, 37- to 42-day embryo the septum is complete and the cloaca is divided into two compartments (Fig. 1-3). The dorsal compartment of the subdivided cloaca is thus the caudal end of the gut, the rectum, while the ventral compartment is the caudal end of the modified allantois, the *urogenital sinus.* From the original tubular shape the sinus comes to be flattened in a dorsoventral diameter.

One of the first alterations of the urogenital sinus is brought about by the junction of the wolffian ducts with the sinus. As we have already noted, tips of the wolffian ducts grow caudally along the mesonephric ridge, swing medially, and abut against the posterior wall of the urogenital sinus, where the lumina of the ducts open into the sinus lumen at about the 7-mm, 5-week stage.

Several major changes in the urogenital sinus take place at precisely this same point. The ends of the müllerian ducts come in and abut against the posterior wall between the two wolffian ducts. The indentation of the sinus wall forms the müllerian tubercle. The sinus epithelial proliferation begins at this point and continues to form the anlage of the vagina. The hymen is formed here. That part of the urogenital sinus above this point subsequently constitutes the urethra (male, prostatic and membranous) while that part below forms the vaginal vestibule (female) or the phallic urethra (male).

Shortly after the wolffian ducts join the urogenital sinus, they produce two dorsally growing buds, the *ureteric buds,* which enlarge into the adjacent mesenchyme to initiate formation of the *metanephric cap* and ultimately the kidney. The stems of the ureteric buds are shifted upward (craniad) along the urogenital sinus to form their own connections with the sinus independent of those of the wolffian ducts with sinus. In due course the ureter is completely separated from its parent, and it com-

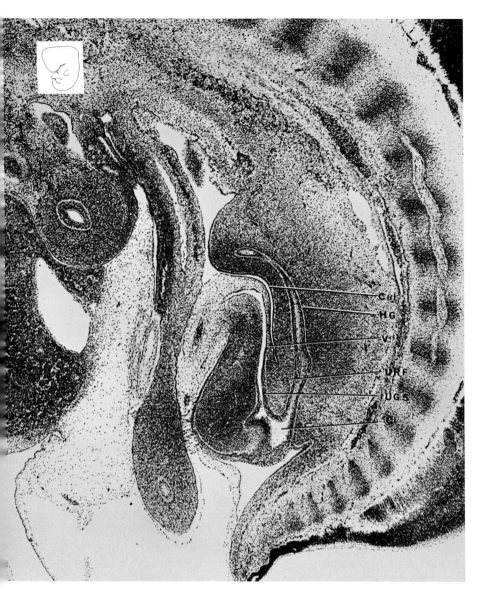

Fig. 1-3. Partition of cloaca. Embryo 8789, 17-1-3; 11.7 mm, 5 weeks. Partition of cloaca (*Cl*) occurs when hindgut (*HG*) joins urogenital sinus (*UGS*), leaves space for urorectal fold (*URF*) which eventually divides sinus, and separates ventral compartment from rectum. Urogenital sinus is continuous with allantois, lower part of which will form bladder (*V*). Cul-de-sac (*Cul*) of celomic cavity is seen as slit between hindgut and urogenital sinus. 15×. (From Dougherty, C. M. *Surgical Pathology of Gynecologic Disease.* New York, Harper & Row, 1968.)

municates with a part of the sinus which is undergoing a bulbous dilation to form the *urinary bladder*. Since the connection is posterolateral,
the two ureters form a triangular area between them and the lower part
of the sinus destined to be internal urethral aperture. Because of the
reinsertion of the lower end of the ureter into the area of the base of the
bladder, one may say that at least a part of this region is constituted
from a wolffian duct derivative. In the female the wolffian duct does not
contribute any other permanent part of the genitourinary system.

It may be observed that the urogenital sinus evolves, by processes just
explained, into certain major structures which are the same in both
sexes above the wolffian ductal junction but into other major structures
different in the two sexes below that junction. The sinus above the
reference region forms the urinary bladder, the trigone, the ureterovesical junctions, and the female urethra in its entirety or the male
prostatic and membranous urethra. A cross-section through the sinus
above shows that it is dorsoventrally flattened, i.e., slit-shaped from side
to side.

Below the point of ductal abutment the urogenital sinus continues
caudad and opens to the outside at the caudal end of the embryo connecting with the external urethral groove. In the male fetus this opening
continues as a median sagittal groove on the under side of the phallus
to its tip and becomes converted into a tube by the fusion of its lateral
edges.

In the female the lower urogenital sinus opens to the outside through
the primitive urogenital opening at the 18-mm, 6½-week stage. This
opening is *not* the site of formation of the hymen. Gradually the lower
sinus increases its anteroposterior (sagittal) diameter, becomes relatively
much shorter, and evolves into the vaginal vestibule. By this succession
of changes the upper sinus in the female performs quite different functions from the lower part. The changes in shape and size take place
abruptly just above the ductal junctions. It is natural, then, to designate
the part of the sinus above as the *pars pelvina* and the part below as the
pars phallica.

The urogenital sinus reaches its maximum undifferentiated form
about the 30- to 50-mm stage of development. The urinary bladder is
easily identifiable, the posterior urethra (male) or entire urethra (female)
can be seen, activity at the site of the müllerian tubercle heralds the start
of the vagina, and a widening opening to the outside presages the formation of the vaginal vestibule. Further development of the sinus sometimes becomes arrested in the intersex individual, and conditions just
described for the early fetus prevail in the newborn infant (persistent
urogenital sinus).

EXTERNAL GENITALIA (4–50 mm)

The first, most obvious, and in most cases only criterion used for judging sex of the human is the configuration of the external genital organs and in particular the presence or absence of a phallus. Ironically, the first judgment may be completely in error, for in certain abnormal cases the external genitalia of the female look more like those of the male, and at a stage of embryonic life the female possesses a definite peniform phallus. One must be familiar, therefore, with the development of the genitalia of both sexes in order to recognize normal and abnormal variations in all stages of formation.

Shortly after formation of the cloacal plate at the tail end of the very early embryo, eminences appear at the sides of the plate and crease it in the midline to form the *cloacal groove*. The area between cloacal plate or groove and body stalk soon forms a low conical eminence representing the earliest visible evidence of the external genital organs and designated as the *genital tubercle*. As the tubercle enlarges the cloacal groove comes to occupy the slope facing the tail, and soon it is divided into two parts by a small transverse bar, the forward *urethral groove* and the rearward *anal pit*. As pointed out by Spaulding, the division of the cloacal groove externally takes place before partition of the cloaca internally, although the external and internal separations are at points which correspond.[18] In the further course of development the urethral groove stretches out along the caudal slope of the tubercle, where measurement of its length may be used as a criterion for determining sex differentiation in the 14- to 15-mm, 5- to 6-week embryo. In males the groove is longer and extends to the apex or glans region of the tubercle, while in the female the groove is shorter, ending at a point below the summit.

The genital tubercle gradually grows more prominent assuming the same phallic configuration in both sexes until about the 25-mm, 7-week stage. In this developmental phase the phallus of the female may be seen to be shaped or curved caudally to a greater degree than is the male phallus. In the further growth period the curvature in the female phallus becomes more and more evident, constituting one of the more easily identifiable characteristics for distinguishing sex of the fetus.

The urethral groove is well outlined on the caudal aspect of the phallus in the 11-mm, 5½-week embryo, its lateral sides bordered by the *urethral folds*. The urethral groove, it will be recalled, is the site at which the urogenital sinus perforates through to form the *primitive urogenital ostium*. This event takes place between the 12-mm and 19-mm stages, at a time when the genital tubercle is undergoing lengthening into phallus but before it is morphologically different in the sexes. The urethral groove thus continues the pars phallica of the urogenital sinus to the outside of the body. The laterally placed urethral folds beginning as small rolls of tissue gradually become more marked until they appear as small leaflets beside the deepened groove. The folds run the length of the groove and end near the undersurface of the glans by coming together in a tapered point. In the male the urethral folds join in the midline and form the median raphe, a landmark which may still be seen in the mature male. Thus joined, the folds convert the urethral groove into the penile urethra and provide an opening well out on the undersurface of the phallus. In the female the urethral folds undergo no additional alterations, but remain as the labia minora of the mature individual.

An important change at about the 16-mm to 19-mm length occurs with the beginning formation of the *labioscrotal folds.* The genital tubercle has already elongated into a somewhat cone-shaped phallus when there appear two rolls of tissue laterally at the base of the tubercle, separated from it by a *lateral phallic groove.* The labioscrotal folds enlarge and extend caudally. In the male they take a position caudal to the penis where they form the scrotum by joining together at the median raphe, a distinctly visible ridge on the scrotum. In the female, after a slow growth period, the labioscrotal folds grow backward in a converging direction and unite behind the urogenital opening as the *posterior commissure* of the vulva (about 40- to 45-mm stage). The folds do not extend forward beyond the phallus, but instead merge with the tissue at the mons and remain slightly divergent, still separated from the base of the phallus. With these changes the female genitalia are formed in essentially their definitive form by about the 50-mm, 11-week stage. The phallus is, of course, the *clitoris,* the urethral folds are the *labia minora,* and the labioscrotal folds the *labia majora.* The urethral groove and pars phallica of the urogenital sinus are in the process of being converted into the much-shortened *vaginal vestibule.*

GONADS (20 mm to postnatal)

The testis of this stage can be easily identified by its fibrous cover, primary (medullary) cords, interstitial cells, and rete cords of the hilar region. There are constrictions at the base of attachment along the urogenital ridge, thus narrowing this portion of the gonad into the *mesorchium* (Fig. 1-4). By the time the fetus is 50 mm long, the testis is well along toward its definitive form. There is a tunica covering, there are

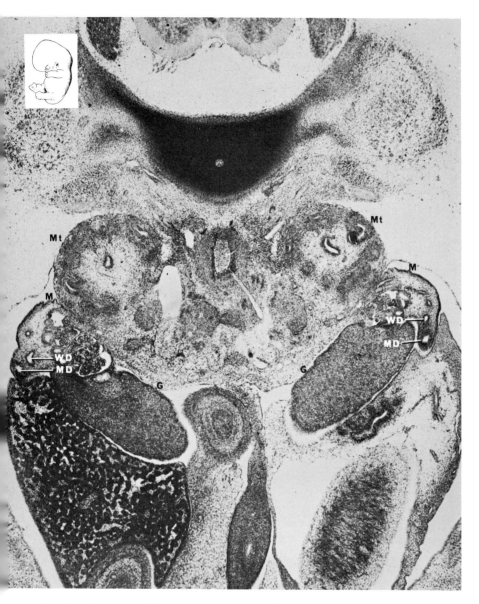

Fig. 1-4. End of indifferent stage. Embryo 7274, 58-3-2; 18 mm, 5½ weeks. Although sex of gonad (G) is still not identifiable by its histologic features, both mesonephros (M) and müllerian ducts (MD) are established. This stage is about the end of sexually indeterminate phase. Mt, metanephros; WD, wolffian duct. 15×. (From Dougherty, C. M. Surgical Pathology of Gynecologic Disease. New York, Harper & Row, 1968.)

seminiferous tubules without lumina, the interstitial cells have differentiated, and the hilar structures are in the process of being formed. There is the start of the great increase in number of interstitial cells, a phenomenon not completely explained by known facts. This multiplication of Leydig cells reaches maximal proportions at about 150 mm, 19 weeks, then decreases from about the 200-mm to the postnatal period. Gonocytes of the embryonic testis become incorporated into the medullary cords, decrease in size, and lose their distinctive appearance. Continued growth of the seminiferous tubules results in their being coiled and crowded. Lumina form within the tubules, and spermatogonia and Sertoli cells may be detected.

By the time the fetus reaches the seventh month and about 240 mm in length, the testes, complete with sperm-carrying apparatus descend into the scrotum through the inguinal canal.

Further development of the ovary takes a longer time, since medullary cords must first be formed and then crowded into the inner part of the organ eventually to disappear due to overgrowth of the newly forming cortex. The ovary at the 20-mm, 7-week stage may be identified by its germinal epithelial cover, masses of ovogonia, absence of prominent sex cords, and more clear-cut cortical-medullary divisions (Fig. 1-5). The early ovary, like the early testis, begins to pendulate from its *mesovarium* formed by constrictions at the attachment to the urogenital ridge. It will be noted that only the middle half to two-thirds of the ridge participates in forming the active ovary, while the cranial and caudal portions become attenuated to form the ovarian and the utero-ovarian ligaments. Limitation of the extent of the ovary is conditioned early when there is a concentration of the migrating gonocytes in the midportion of the gonadal ridge.

Following the first changes which differentiate ovary from testis, the ovary continues on a rather prolonged growth period. The bulk is increased by proliferation of the epithelial cover, forming an outer cellular zone. By this mechanism the *ovarian cortex* is superimposed, as it were, on the medullary portion. The primary sex cords with some of the gonocytes are carried into the medullary region, some of them disappearing and some remaining for variable lengths of time. In studying serial sections of fetal ovaries of graduated ages, Forbes noted that the medullary cords disappeared from the ovary between the ages of 280 and 350 mm.[4] He found none remaining in postnatal ovaries. It is of interest that Meyer believed that medullary cords persisted occasionally in the adult organ and that in a few of these they gave rise to masculinizing ovarian tumors, specifically the arrhenoblastoma.[12]

Soon after arrival in the gonadal blastema (8 mm, $4\frac{1}{2}$ weeks) the

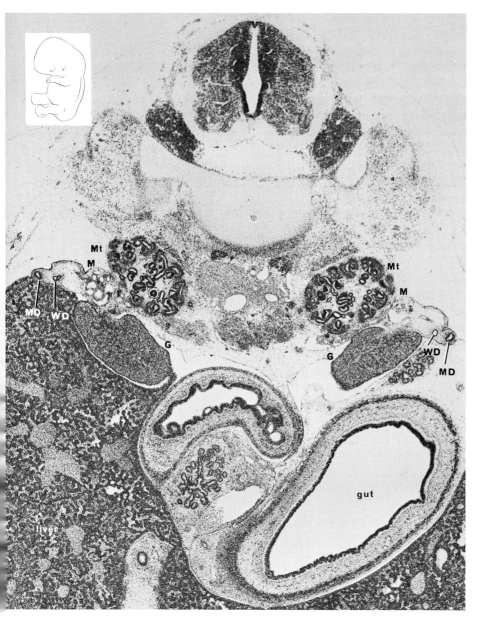

Fig. 1-5. Beginning of differentiated stage. Embryo 8553, 89-3-2; 22 mm, 6 weeks. Gonad (G) may be identified as ovary. Metanephros (Mt) is well along in its formation, and both ducts, mesonephric (WD) and müllerian (MD), are clearly seen on each side. Plane of this section is caudal to main portion of mesonephros (M), part of which may be seen on both sides. 15×. (From Dougherty, C. M. Surgical Pathology of Gynecologic Disease. New York, Harper & Row, 1968.)

gonocytes undergo rather sustained multiplication, some of them being incorporated in the epithelial sex cords, others remaining within the mesenchymal stroma. During this period the sex cells tend to be less conspicuous than they were on first migration to the gonad, being somewhat smaller. Older embryologists, noting this change, explained it by hypothesizing that the larger cells were "genitaloid," or that the first germ cells disappeared from the ovary to be followed by a new crop of germ cells.

The most prominent feature of the ovary of the 17-week, 125-mm fetus is the large number of ovocytes. The deeper ones, those near the hilar or medullary region, may be seen to be surrounded by smaller dark somatic cells, the granulosa cells of *primitive follicles.* The cortical region of the ovary is plainly separate from the hilum from which small blood vessels run radially to the periphery of the organ, dividing cortex into segments. The more superficial of the ovocytes appear in small clusters or "families," probably the result of successive divisions of these cells.

Continued development of the ovary takes place by quantitative rather than qualitative changes (Fig. 1-6). Near term and in the newborn female there is evidence of follicular development, and it is not unusual to find small follicle cysts just beneath the surface. From term to about 2 years postnatally there is a drastic reduction in the total number of ova in the ovary, the decrease probably accomplished by follicular atresia. Estimates of the total number of ova within the ovary at different periods of development show the rapid increase and subsequent decrease in cells: [1,2,7,21]

Embryo, 4.2 mm	1,366
Fetus, 100–200 mm	5,000,000–6,000,000
Newborn infant	5,000,000–6,000,000
Adolescent girl	500,000
Mature young adult	159,000

WOLFFIAN DUCT (30 mm to postnatal)

After reaching the urogenital sinus and providing guides for the course of the müllerian duct, the wolffian ducts continue their development or become vestigial, depending upon whether they are or are not influenced by the testis (Figs. 1-7 and 1-8). Apparently this influence operates locally, as may be seen in an interesting experiment of nature. In the normal embryo both members of the pair of ducts evolve in the same manner, but in certain hermaphroditic states where one gonad is testis

Fig. 1-6. (*A–F*, pages 21–23). Development of the female germ cells. *A*. Embryo 836, 10-2-1; 4mm. Primitive germ cells in yolk sac entoderm. Large clear cells (gonocytes) are among epithelial cells which line hindgut. Although tentative recognition of germ cells has been reported in early ovum, this stage represents earliest period at which reasonably accurate identification of gonocyte has been made. 75×. *B*. Embryo 7889, 4-2-3; 4.2 mm. Gonocytes, large cells having clear cytoplasm, are seen in mesenchyme of mesentery during short migration from yolk sac to gonadal ridge. 335×.

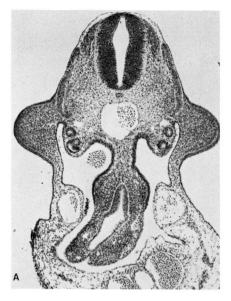

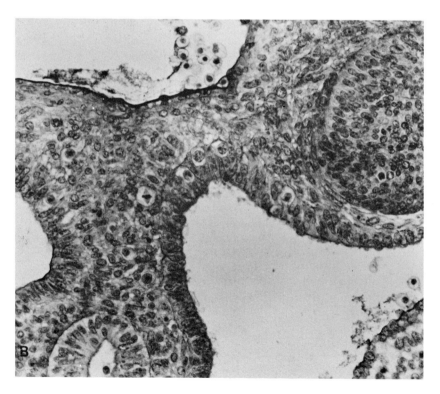

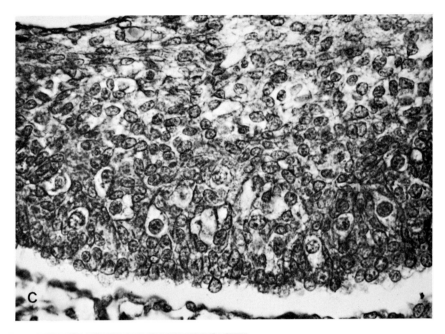

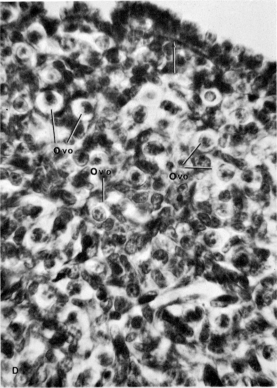

Fig. 1-6. C. Embryo 8101, 30-3-7; 13 mm. Ovogonia within ovarian cortex. Large clear germ cells occupy positions in germinal epithelium and mesenchymal cortex of gonadal ridge. 450×. D. Embryo H-14, 85-1-2; 26 mm. Large numbers of ovogonia (*Ovo*) in ovary. Germ cells multiply greatly after arriving in epithelium and mesenchyme of gonad. This stage and this germ cell may be time and place of appearance of tumorogenic factors or actual tumors of germ cell origin. Germinal epithelium several cells thick is marked off by basement membrane (arrow). 480×.

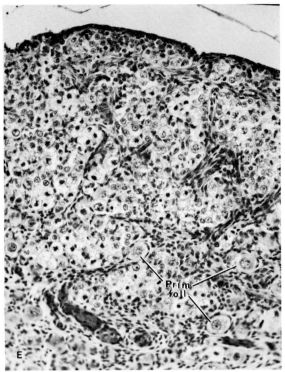

Fig. 1-6. *E.* Embryo 7774, 9-3-4; 221 mm. Germ cell maturation in ovary. Ovary is crowded with ovogonia, many of which have matured into ovocytes and become surrounded by layer of stromal cells, forming primary follicles (*Prim foll*). Spindle cells of ovarian cortical stroma may be found between germ cells. Germ cells in mitosis are visible evidence that these cells are in process of multiplication. 200×. (*D* & *E* from Dougherty, C. M. *Surgical Pathology of Gynecologic Disease.* New York, Harper & Row, 1968.) *F.* Embryo 12-12A, 8-3-6; 331 mm, 9 months. Primary ovocytes are surrounded by progranulosa or granulosa cells. Germ cells in medulla of gonad have disappeared. Cortex is crowded with primordial follicles. 100×.

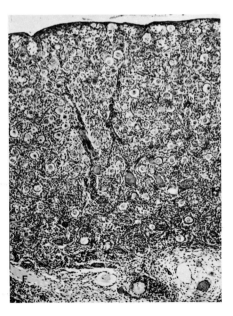

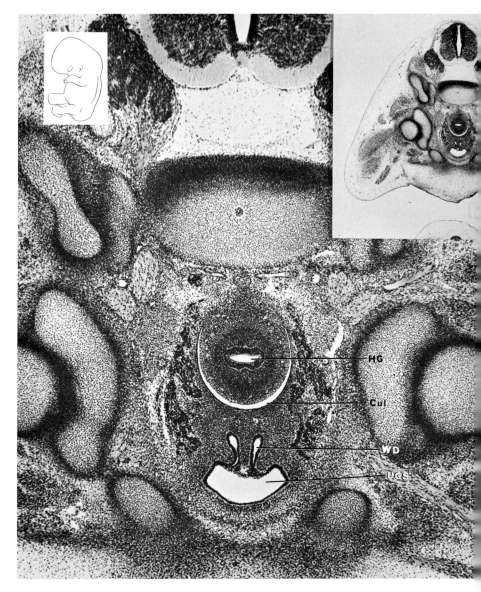

Fig. 1-7. Mesonephric ducts join urogenital sinus. Embryo 8553, 95-2-1; 22 mm, 6 weeks. Cross-section near caudal end demonstrates junction of mesonephric ducts (*WD*) with dorsal wall of urogenital sinus (*UGS*). Hindgut (*HG*) lies behind this confluens and is separated by a caudal extension of celomic cavity, pouch of Douglas (*Cul*). Müllerian ducts have not extended this far caudally yet. 15×. (From Dougherty, C. M. *Surgical Pathology of Gynecologic Disease*. New York, Harper & Row, 1968.)

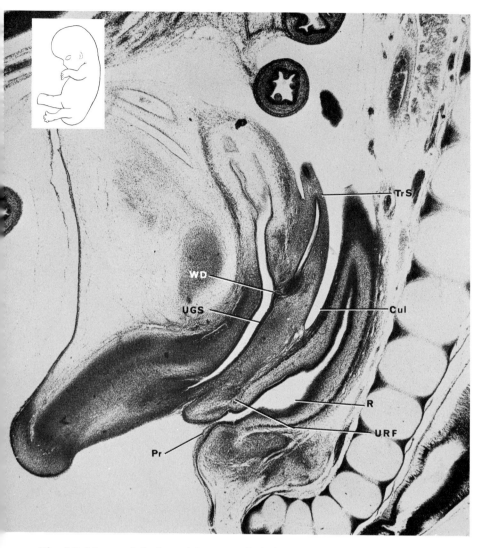

Fig. 1-8. Mesonephric ducts join urogenital sinus. Embryo 5422, 32-1; 27 mm, 6½ weeks. Caudal region is depicted in this sagittal section just off midline and shows mesonephric duct (*WD*) opening into urogenital sinus (*UGS*). This point is used as arbitrary boundary mark between vesicourethral portion cephalad and definitive urogenital sinus (pars pelvina) caudally. Rectum (*R*) has already been partitioned by urorectal fold (*URF*) extending all the way to cloacal membrane, and proctodeum (*Pr*) has opened. Caudal extension of celomic cavity forms cul-de-sac of Douglas (*Cul*). Transverse septum (*TrS*) of pelvis is seen in cross-section. 15×. (From Dougherty, C. M. *Surgical Pathology of Gynecologic Disease.* New York, Harper & Row, 1968.)

and the other is ovary, one wolffian duct develops into vas deferens and epididymis while the other undergoes atrophy.

In the male embryo the wolffian duct retains its connections with the mesonephric tubules, and when the testis enlarges and differentiates, duct and tubules form the major part of the sperm-collecting apparatus. The cranial end of the ductal apparatus migrates through the inguinal canal with the testis to its destination in the scrotum, while the caudal end of the duct keeps its relation with the urogenital sinus, eventually emptying into the prostatic urethra.

In the female the wolffian duct and tubules not only stop growing but actually undergo involution along with the mesonephros when the ovary differentiates until, in the 60- to 100-mm female fetus they constitute vestigial remnants. With the exception of the ureter and kidney pelvis, no part of the wolffian apparatus remains functional in the adult. Vestigial remnants may be seen in the mesovarium where some 10–20 of the caudalmost tubules appear as tiny threads, and in the mesosalpinx and occasionally in the substance of the cervix where microscopic residues of the duct persist.

MÜLLERIAN DUCTS (32 mm to postnatal)

In contrast to the rapid development of the wolffian ducts, that of the müllerian ducts is slow. The two ducts growing caudally reach the dorsal wall of the urogenital sinus in an oblique angle at a point between the more laterally placed wolffian ducts (Figs. 1-9 and 1-10). There they rest but do not open into the sinus. While the sinus epithelium begins to proliferate, the two müllerian ducts fuse together into a single-channeled genital canal, usually called the *uterovaginal canal* (Fig. 1-11). The intervening septum is dissolved from caudal to cranial direction starting at a variable time around the 42-mm stage. A thin strip of mesenchymal tissue intervenes between sinus wall and müllerian ductal ends. The tip is still composed of a solid mass of müllerian epithelium, at this time clearly distinct from sinus epithelium. With the exception of the tip, the uterovaginal canal is lined with a single layer of müllerian epithelium.

Two noticeable bulges of mesenchymal cells surround the regions of the future corpus uteri and future cervix uteri, while smaller aggregations are found around the isthmic and vaginal portions. The fundus region of the uterus is notched in a wide V-shape where the two ducts join. Differentiation of smooth muscle from the undifferentiated mesenchymal cells is said to begin at about 170 mm, 20½ weeks, and to be substantially complete at 210 mm, 24½ weeks.[9] The eventual rounding

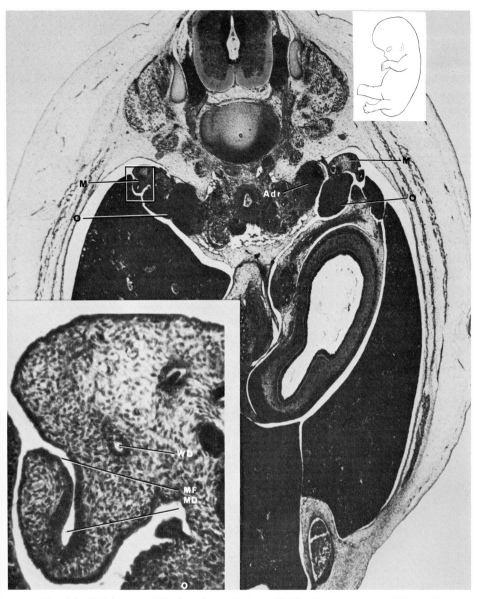

Fig. 1-9. Origin of müllerian duct. Embryo H-14, 85-1-2; 26 mm, 6½ weeks. Müllerian funnel (*MF*) is a groove-like invagination of celomic lining near cephalic pole of mesonephros (*M*). From this starting point, müllerian duct (*MD*) grows back all the way to caudal region where it ends against urogenital sinus. Wolffian duct is medial (*WD*). Close relation of cranial end of ovary (*O*) and fetal adrenal cortex (*Adr*) is demonstrated in this section. 12× (*Inset,* 240×). (From Dougherty, C. M. *Surgical Pathology of Gynecologic Disease.* New York, Harper & Row, 1968.)

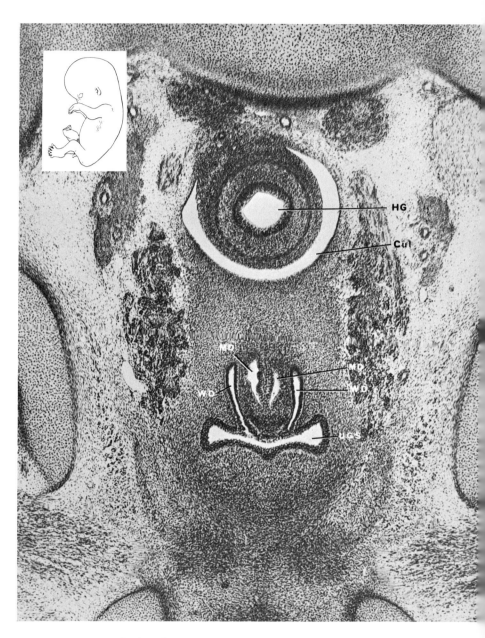

Fig. 1-10. Müllerian ducts reach urogenital sinus. Embryo 6573, 74-3-2; 31.5 mm, 7 weeks. Mesonephric ducts (*WD*) open into urogenital sinus (*UGS*), while müllerian ducts (*MD*) occupy medial position in this area and do not yet open into sinus. Hindgut (*HG*) and pouch of Douglas (*Cul*) are behind urogenital sinus. 45×. (From Dougherty, C. M. *Surgical Pathology of Gynecologic Disease.* New York, Harper & Row, 1968.)

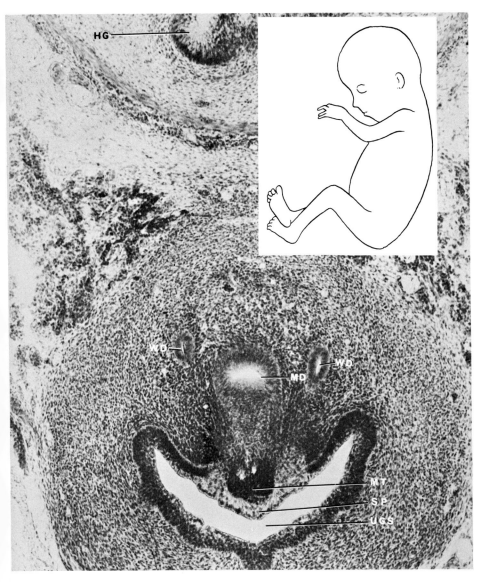

Fig. 1-11. Formation of müllerian tubercle. Embryo 6017, 4-5-5; 60 mm, 12 weeks. At point where müllerian ducts come back to urogenital sinus (*UGS*), they are fused into single canal (*MD*) and end in dense aggregate of mesenchymal cells. Solid proliferation of posterior wall of sinus in immediate region where ducts abut sinus is müllerian tubercle (*MT*). Mound of sinus epithelium (*SP*) is composed of differentiated type of cell, probably forerunner of vaginal epithelium. Oblique sections through mesonephric ducts (*WD*) are seen lateral to fused müllerian ducts. The hindgut (*HG*) is dorsal. 100×. (From Dougherty, C. M. *Surgical Pathology of Gynecologic Disease*. New York, Harper & Row, 1968.)

out of the fundal contour results from the thickening of the muscular wall of the corpus uteri.

The endocervical epithelium begins to assume the characteristics of mucous type beginning at the twenty-fourth week.[9] At this time and for some time later the subepithelial stromal tissue of the cervix and that of the corpus are composed of undifferentiated spindle cells all very similar. The epithelium of the corpus is of a tall columnar type but without the clear cytoplasm of the mucous variety of epithelium beginning to appear in the endocervix.

When the development of the uterus reaches about the 150-mm stage, there are a few shallow simple tubular glands in the corpus and quite a number in the endocervix. The predominance of cervical glands persists long after the postnatal period.

UROGENITAL SINUS (50 mm to postnatal)

In the embryo of about 65-mm, $11\frac{1}{2}$-week size one may see an active proliferation forming paired eminences of epithelium of the posterior wall of the urogenital sinus in the region formerly occupied by the müllerian tubercle. These masses are the *sinovaginal bulbs*[13] or *dorsolateral proliferations*,[3] forerunner of the vagina. Intense activity and growth take place in both types of epithelia, resulting in two changes: solidification of the lumen of the uterovaginal canal and relative lengthening of the cellular plate, cord, or ribbon, from which the future vagina is fashioned. One author described the process of solidification of the lumen of the uterovaginal canal as a "conversion of (müllerian) columnar to stratified epithelium" which "continues cranially until the transition between the two types becomes abrupt, a point which marks the junction of cervical and vaginal epithelium in the cervical canal." [10] Other investigators found a proliferation of darkly stained cells of the dorsal sinus wall which displaces the müllerian epithelium in a cranial direction to form a solid cord. This cord subsequently becomes canalized as the entire vagina.[20] In a more recent study of the origin of the vagina, yet another author noted proliferation of the dorsal sinus epithelium from two lateral foci near the ends of the wolffian ducts and from an intermediate focus between the two lateral regions, all three of which elements combine to displace all müllerian epithelium from the length of the vagina.[3] Thus, in the opinion of one of these investigators the upper part of the vagina develops from the müllerian ducts and the lower part from the sinus epithelium in the ratio of about four-fifths to one-fifth.[10] In the view of the others, the vagina in its entirety comes from the proliferated sinus epithelium.[3, 13, 20] The junction of sinus and müllerian epithelia is at the level of the external cervical os.

In summary, the vagina has its beginning in the 65-mm, 12-week fetus as solidification of the caudal müllerian genital canal and an upgrowth of sinus epithelium from the dorsal wall of the urogenital sinus. The sinus upgrowth forms a ribbon or cord which displaces the müllerian epithelium craniad at least part and probably all the way to the cervix, forming the anlage of the future hollow tubular vagina.

Growth and development of the vaginal ribbon continues slowly, with stratification and proliferation of cells until relatively large bulbous formations of multilayered epithelium may be seen in the 125-mm fetus. With continued maturation of the epithelium, there is beginning desquamation of the central cells and creation of a new lumen. Canalization proceeds from caudal to cranial direction. The lumen is complete in the vagina and is separated from the cervical canal in the 162-mm fetus by only a small plug of cells.

The epithelial lining of the vagina is many layers thick, with a darkly stained basal layer and glycogen-bearing superficial layers similar to the type seen in the gravid adult female.

When the epithelium of the vaginal ribbon differentiates and becomes glycogenated, it traces around the vaginal portion of the cervix anteriorly and posteriorly where alae outline the shape of the *vaginal fornices* (150 mm, 18 weeks). When the main portion of the vaginal epithelium becomes canalized, the fornices also develop clefts, which complete the definitive form of the upper vagina, there being a multicellular layer of vaginal epithelium on the cervical face as well as on the vaginal side.

Elongation and thickening of the epithelial mass forming the vaginal anlage reach enormous proportions from about the 100- to 150-mm, 16- to 18-week stage of growth. That end which joins cranially with the vaginal portion of the cervix is limited by the fornices, while the caudal end rests against the dorsal wall of the pars phallica of the urogenital sinus at an acute angle. Two important structures are thereby brought nearer to definitive shapes. The *hymen* is formed as a lunate infolding transversely across the dorsal wall of the phallic portion of the urogenital sinus, a folding caused by the pressure of caudal growth of the large mass of vaginal epithelium by the 120- to 150-mm stage. Thus, the hymen is formed at some distance from the urogenital ostium, the first opening of the urinary and genital tracts to the outside of the body. It eventually comes to occupy a position very near the external genitalia when the pars phallica changes shape and length in forming the *vaginal vestibule*.

The *urethra* assumes a relation with the newly forming vaginal anlage similar to its relation in the fully developed state. It will be recalled that the ureters, the urinary bladder, and the trigone are formed at a relatively early stage, 15 mm, 5¾ weeks, compared with the formation of the vagina and müllerian system. In the female the entire urethra comes from that part of the urogenital sinus (pars pelvina) between the bladder and the müllerian tubercle, later the site of confluence of the vaginal lumen and the sinus lumen. As the vaginal cord becomes more prominent, it slowly approaches a longitudinal relation closer to parallel with the urogenital sinus, until, in the 160-mm, 19-week fetus its position is next to the urethra and a "septum" is seen in the place where the "anterior" (ventral) vaginal wall of the fully developed vagina is located. The urethra is flanked in its midsection by many small diverticular glands dorsally and laterally, the forerunners of the prostate in the male and the periurethral glands in the female.

By the time the fetus has reached the 160-mm, 19-week period, the pars phallica of the urogenital sinus has evolved into a foreshortened conduit with a long sagittal diameter. A relatively great increase in size of the vagina has brought its opening just inside the folds of the external genitalia and, since the vagina has assumed a parallel position with the urethra, vaginal and urethral openings are together in a ventral-caudal arrangement. In the full course of this development, then, the pars phallica of the urogenital sinus progresses from a long simple tube to a short wide sagittal cleft in the base of which are the separate openings of the urinary and genital tracts. Named the vestibule of the vagina, it could as readily and perhaps more accurately be called the urethrovaginal vestibule.

In the 40-mm, 10-week fetus the widened and shortened pars phallica may be seen to have two small lateral glandular structures connected to it by short ducts. These are the *Bartholin glands,* the female equivalent of the male bulbourethral glands (Cowper's). At first located a short distance from the focal point of activity of the sinus beside the sinus epithelial upgrowth of the future vagina, the glands eventually come to a position just caudal to the hymen, where they may be found in the fully developed individual.

EXTERNAL GENITALIA (50 mm to postnatal)

Changes in the male external genitalia just preceding this period of development (40–50 mm) are important in shaping them into the definitive form. The coronal sulcus has separated the glans from the remainder of the phallus, the urethral folds have fused in the midline (median raphe) forming the penile urethra, the labioscrotal folds have migrated to a site caudal to the penis to constitute the scrotum, and space between the anus and urogenital opening has greatly increased. In the female, though they are not so extensive, the changes tend to parallel those of the male, and the genitalia gradually assume the definitive form also. The glans clitoridis is outlined by the coronal sulcus, the urethral folds bordering the urethral meatus and the vaginal orifice assume the role of labia minora, and the labioscrotal swellings enclose the inner structures named.

Up until this stage of development the phalluses of the male and the female fetuses are of approximately the same length, but in the female the caudal curvature is distinctive. While only a portion of the female phallus is masked by the large labia, the male phallus is made to seem shorter by the height of the scrotal bulge at its base.

At the 50-mm stage the glans of both penis and clitoris are conspicuous as a bulbous, unsheathed terminal part. Between this period and the 100-mm stage, the prepuce is gradually formed by folds from the shaft which extend to cover the whole glans. The prepuce is said to form more rapidly in the male than in the female, since in the female several folds of skin are involved in the process.[18]

SUPPORTING STRUCTURES

Certain supporting structures, ligaments of aggregated connective tissue, are formed from the structures adjacent to and connected with the gonads and genital ducts. Homologies of these supports of the two sexes can readily be seen.

The *mesovarium* makes its appearance when there is longitudinal constriction between the mesonephros and the genital portion of the urogenital ridge. When the fetus reaches the 20- to 25-mm stage, the constriction has produced a well-defined web-like pedicle by which the ovary hangs in the celomic cavity. Vascular development is evident through the mesentery of the ovary and the hilum. At this early stage of development the mesovarium and *mesorchium* are closely similar, each being affixed to the respective gonad at the hilum, continuous with the medulla and containing a few of the medullary structures.

When the ovary eventually assumes its pelvic position, the mesovarium reaches from uterine fundus to the dorsolateral pelvic wall, a location which is foretold by the original position of the urogenital ridge. The mesovarium contains vestigial remnants of mesonephric tubules from the midportion of the mesonephros and the longitudinal vestigial mesonephric duct.

The *suspensory ligament* of the ovary, extending from the cephalic

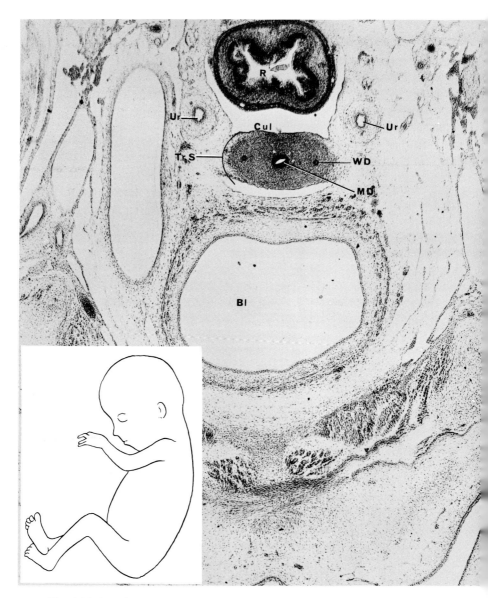

Fig. 1-12. Development of transverse septum. Embryo 6017, 7-3-4; 60 mm, 12 weeks. Fused müllerian ducts (*MD*) in center and paired mesonephric ducts (*WD*) laterally are seen in dense condensation of mesenchyme forming transverse pelvic septum (*TrS*), forerunner of broad ligament and corpus uteri. Large urinary bladder (*Bl*) is ventral to transverse septum from which it is separated by anterior (ventral) cul-de-sac. Dorsally situated rectosigmoid (*R*) is separated by posterior cul-de-sac of Douglas (*Cul*). Farther laterally, ureters (*Ur*) are seen. 30×. (From Dougherty, C. M. *Surgical Pathology of Gynecologic Disease*. New York, Harper & Row, 1968.)

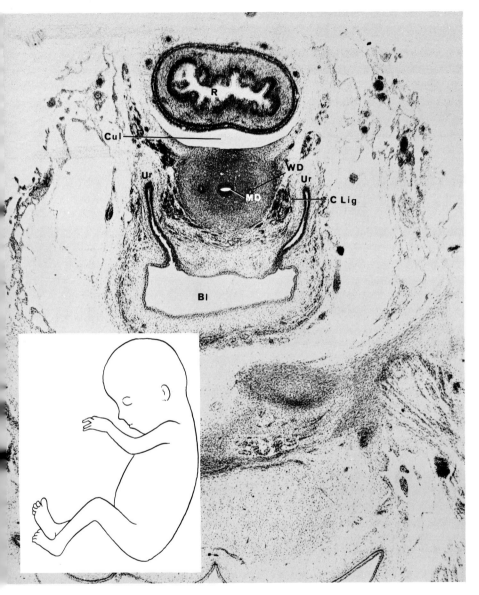

Fig. 1-13. Mesenchymal elements constitute supporting structures. Embryo 6017, 8-4-1; 60 mm, 12 weeks. Ureters (*Ur*) join urinary bladder (*Bl*), lined by type of transitional epithelium. Cervicouterine stroma is condensed around fused müllerian ducts (*MD*) and supported by cardinal ligaments (*C Lig*). Mesonephric ducts (*WD*), no longer prominent, are still present in lateral position. Hindgut (*R*) and cul-de-sac of Douglas (*Cul*) are dorsal to genital apparatus. 30×. (From Dougherty, C. M. *Surgical Pathology of Gynecologic Disease*. New York, Harper & Row, 1968.)

pole of the ovary, is formed from the anterior one-fourth of the urogenital ridge. In the mature female there are no epithelial elements or residues within this structure, but the ovarian cortex sometimes appears to extend outward, partly covering and blending into the fibrous tissue of the ligament, thus proving that it was formerly a related type of tissue.

The *utero-ovarian ligament* together with the round ligament are derived from the caudal end of the urogenital ridge. The homologous part in the male is the *gubernaculum testis,* attached to the caudal pole of the testis. At first one continuous ligament, the utero-ovarian and round ligaments come to be apparently separate when a knuckle is incorporated into the developing myometrium and the two assume slightly different relations with the uterus. The round ligament, in coursing through the inguinal canal and ending within the subcutaneous tissue of the labia majora, traces in the female the path by which the gubernaculum testis in the male guides the descending testis into place within the scrotum.

The *broad ligament* with the fallopian tube attached along its border is first seen in the early embryo as the transverse septum of the pelvis (Figs. 1-12 and 1-13). It carries first the wolffian duct, then later the müllerian duct. After the formation of the uterus and tubes from the müllerian ducts, the lateral wings of the transverse septum thin out into little more than two layers of peritoneum. The vestigial remnant of the wolffian duct may be identified running parallel to the tube between the leaves of the broad ligament.

The *uterosacral* ligaments are formed by folds of peritoneum and fibrous tissue in the pouch of Douglas just lateral to the hindgut. The folds are anchored ventrally to a portion of the transverse septum of the pelvis representing the future cervix. Dorsally the folds attach to the pelvic wall in the region of the lateral borders of the sacrum at about its third or fourth segment.

REFERENCES

1. BAKER, T. G. A quantitative and cytological study of germ cells in human ovaries. *Proc R Soc Lond 158:*417, 1963.
2. BLOCK, E. Quantitative morphological investigations of the follicular system in women. *Acta Anat 14:*108, 1952.
3. BULMER, D. The development of the human vagina. *J Anat 91:*490, 496, 1957.
4. FORBES, T. R. On the fate of the medullary cords of the human ovary. *Contrib Embryol 188:*11, 1942.
5. FUSS, A. Uber extraegionare Geschlechtszellen bein einem menschlichen Embryo von 4 Wochen. *Anat Anz 39:*407, 1911.
6. GILLMAN, J. The development of the gonads in man, with a consideration of the role of fetal endocrines and the histogenesis of ovarian tumors. *Contrib Embryol 210:*85, 107, 1948.

7. GREENHILL, J. P. *Obstetrics,* ed. 13. Philadelphia, Saunders, 1965, p. 34.

8. HAMLETT, G. W. D. Primordial germ cells in 4.5 mm. human embryo. *Anat Rec 61:*273, 1935.

9. HUNTER, R. H. Observations on the development of the human female genital tract. *Contrib Embryol 129:*101, 103, 1930.

10. KOFF, A. K. Development of the vagina in the human fetus. *Contrib Embryol 140:*61, 73, 1933.

11. McKAY, D. G., HERTIG, A. T., ADAMS, E. C., and DANZIGER, S. Histochemical observations on the germ cells of the human embryo. *Anat Rec 117:*201, 1953.

12. MEYER, R. The pathology of some special ovarian tumors and their relation to sex characteristics. *Am J Obstet Gynecol 22:*697, 1931.

13. MEYER, R. Zur Frage der Entwicklung der menschlichen Vagina, Teil IV. *Arch Gynaekol 165:*504, 1938.

14. MORRIS, J. M., and SCULLY, R. E. *Endocrine Pathology of the Ovary.* St. Louis, Mosby, 1958, p. 22.

15. PINKERTON, J. H. M., McKAY, D. G., ADAMS, E. C., and HERTIG, A. T. Development of the human ovary: A study using histochemical technics. *Obstet Gynecol 18:*152, 1961.

16. POTTER, E. *Pathology of the Fetus and the Newborn.* Chicago, Year Book, 1952, p. 14.

17. SELLMANN, A. H., and DOUGHERTY, C. M. The development of the female genital tract. *Ann NY Acad Sci 142:*576, 1967.

18. SPAULDING, M. H. The development of the external genitalia in the human embryo. *Contrib Embryol 13:*69, 83, 1210, 1921.

19. TURNER, C. D. Special mechanisms in anomalies of sex differentiation. *Am J Obstet Gynecol 90:*1211–1212, 1964.

20. VILAS, E. Uber die Entwicklung der menschlichen Scheide. *Z Anat Entwicklungsgesch 98:*263, 1932.

21. WITSCHI, E. Embryology of the Ovary. In Grady, H. G., and Smith, D. E. (eds.) *The Ovary.* Baltimore, Williams & Wilkins, 1963, pp. 1–10.

22. WITSCHI, E. Migration of the germ cells of human embryos from the yolk sac to the primitive gonadal folds. *Contrib Embryol 209:*69–80, 1948.

23. WOLL, E., HERTIG, A. T., SMITH, G. V. S., and JOHNSON, L. C. The ovary in endometrial carcinoma. *Am J Obstet Gynecol 56:*617, 1948.

Chapter Two

Anomalies in the Fetus

A. H. Sellmann and Cary M. Dougherty

Are the kinds and extent of anomalous changes in the fetus different from those found in the newborn or the young adult? Are developmental defects of the genital organs of sufficient gravity to initiate the process of abortion or previable premature delivery? Are these errors usually associated with others of greater severity in other systems in the production of pregnancy loss? Does the successful treatment of threatened abortion contribute to the salvage of a female with a defective genital system? Are there clues to be found in the examination of abortuses which could lead to a better understanding of the causes of malformations of the genital tract in the female?

ANOMALIES IN THE EARLY STAGES OF MAMMALIAN REPRODUCTION

Much information pertinent to these questions regarding human development has been learned from the study of similar problems in other mammals. Amazing parallels have been found.

Studies in comparative embryology have proved that developmental defects in certain mammalian progeny date from the earliest period of development. These findings suggest that in the species studied the rate of reproductive loss is higher than was previously suspected, since a defect occurring at an extremely early age is associated with loss of the entire conceptus rather than malformation of one system or organ.

38

Corner, studying lethal anomalies in the embryonic pig, concluded that there was a loss of some 30 per cent of offspring from the time of fertilization to birth, most of which occurred in the early stages of cleavage and implantation.[5] A similar condition of ovular loss in the very early stages of gestation was found in rhesus monkeys.[6, 12] The major part of the wastage occurred in the first few days or weeks following fertilization.

A far from perfect gross fertility rate has also been demonstrated in the case of wild rabbits, among which Brambell found about 43 per cent reproductive loss mostly occurring in the early part of gestation,[1] and in the case of rats, in which Frazer noted a 20 per cent loss of implanted ova.[7]

Thus, it is evident that developmental defects may appear with the very first cleavage of the ovum and be of such magnitude as to cause loss of the conceptus. It is open to speculation just how serious these early defects must be to produce ovular loss or how mild to effect no damage at all to the offspring. One would be inclined to reason that there are none so mild that they do not leave their mark in one system or another.

ANOMALIES IN THE EARLY HUMAN OVUM

The Hertig-Rock Studies

Because of the publication of reports of the careful scientific studies by Hertig and associates, the early stages of human embryogenesis, both normal and abnormal, are now documented.[8] Using a technique of rinsing with saline the fallopian tubes and endometrial cavities of surgical specimens, Hertig recovered 8 free-lying fertilized ova. By inspection of the lining of the uterus in other cases he found 26 implanted ova. Of the 34 specimens, 21 were normal and 13 were considered abnormal.

Abnormal Uterine Ova

The 9 implanted ova judged to be abnormal were described by Hertig as follows: 1 ovum with syncytiotrophoblast only, 1 ovum with poor trophoblast and no embryo, 1 ovum with relatively good trophoblast but no chorionic cavity, 3 ova with variable degrees of trophoblastic hypoplasia, 2 ova showing shallow implantation, and 1 specimen whose only abnormality was a maloriented germ disc.[8] It may be presumed that the majority of these ova would have aborted had the uterus remained in place, but it is not certain that all would have done so. Very likely some would have developed further only to show some degree of abnormality later.

Implantation Site

In this study more normal ova were found implanted in the posterior wall of the uterus, while more abnormal ova were implanted in the anterior wall. All 26 implanted ova were within the upper half of the uterine corpus.

Condition of the Endometrium

Hertig found the endometrium to be completely normal in the uteri where the 9 abnormal ova were discovered. The hormonal effect upon the uterine mucosa was not only morphologically normal but also of a degree in phase with the schedule of development of the progestational pattern. Thus, "the endometria gave no morphologic evidence of or reason for such abnormalities." [8]

Condition of the Corpus Luteum

Hertig found that the early abnormal ova were associated with abnormal corpora lutea. These structures all manifested a poor secretory quality, possibly due to the inadequate trophoblastic stimulation of malformed ova. Since a defective trophoblast might be morphologically normal but functionally abnormal, morphologic study would not necessarily demonstrate the defect. But whether there is a functional abnormality or not, Hertig's findings implicate, on a morphologic basis, the poor quality of the corpora lutea as a probable cause of abortion. Further speculation along this line leads to the conclusion that administration of exogenous progestins to the woman with an abnormal ovum and inadequate corpus luteum might salvage a defective offspring. Given the high percentage of implanted abnormal ova encountered by Hertig (9 of 26), the risk of saving such an egg is significant.

Causes of Anomalies

Although no reference is made to the antecedent causes of abnormalities of the early ova under study, the authors must have felt that at least some were of genetic origin while others were due to environmental elements, as emphasized by the older embryologists. The implication is clear, however, that prevention of abortion by administration of hormones at an early stage of gestation is ill advised because it may promote either retention of a bad egg or damage of a good egg.

ANOMALIES IN THE EMBRYO AND FETUS

Study of Pathologic Ova by Mall and Meyer

By far the most exhaustive study of pathologic human ova, embryos, and fetuses ("cyemata") was carried out and recorded by Mall and

Meyer.[14] These authors reviewed and analyzed the conceptuses classified as pathologic in the first 1000 accessions to the collections of the Department of Embryology of the Carnegie Institution of Washington. In this collection of specimens contributed by interested practitioners there was a preponderance of young embryos and of cyemata having visible abnormalities.

Definitions

Their specimens were classified in one of two great divisions—normal and pathologic. Normal embryos and fetuses were all those which were normal in form even though some of them had localized anomalies or were enclosed in diseased chorions.[14] "The basis for grading specimens was wholly gross morphologic." [14] A sharply defined, well-formed, white embryo, with blood vessels shining through its transparent tissues, was considered normal. If it were partly stunted and opaque or disintegrating, it was considered pathologic. Among all the abortuses studied, Mall found 560 normal and 313 pathologic specimens (uterine).

Classification of Pathologic Ova

Mall's pathologic division comprised seven classes of specimens subdivided largely on the basis of the degree of destruction of the ovum or embryo. In Groups 1 through 3 the embryo or fetus was missing entirely. These groups were described as (1) chorionic villi only, (2) chorionic vesicle wholly devoid of contents, and (3) chorion and amnion only. In describing these specimens as pathologic, Mall stated: "This does not imply, however, that they themselves necessarily are diseased. In fact many (most?) of these specimens probably were the victims of accident, interference, or untoward conditions, and hence may have been entirely normal at the time of death." [14]

In the other four categories of pathologic ova Mall placed embryos and fetuses which were more likely developmentally defective: (4) nodular fetus, (5) cylindrical fetus, (6) stunted fetus, and (7) fetus compressus. In these last four groups the fetuses were greatly abnormal and incapable of developing into a form even remotely resembling the normal. Presumably the ova which produced these fetal monstrosities were indeed bad eggs. The study of specimens such as these is primarily the interest of the embryologist as a basic scientist.

Sex Incidence in Abortions

Schultz defined the sex ratio at conception, or sex ratio of the fertilized ova, as the primary sex ratio; that existing at the time of birth as the secondary sex ratio; and the number of males per 100 females at the time of maturity (adulthood) as the tertiary sex ratio.[19] Using vital statistics and a composite calculation based on a review of estimates offered by other authors, Schultz concluded: "From these quotations it would seem most probable, on a rough average, that out of every 100 fertilized ova only 78, or even less, develop to term, the remainder being aborted." [19] Like later investigators, Schultz found that the frequency of abortions is greatest in the first 3 months of pregnancy. He noted, in summary, "that more males . . . are conceived; that at certain periods of pregnancy the relative mortality of males exceeds that of females by as much as one fourth; . . . and that this, in connection with the very high intrauterine mortality, . . . serves to lower the primary sex ratio considerably throughout prenatal life." [14]

Anomalies by Organ Systems

Among Mall's 333 pathologic uterine abortuses, 38 specimens exhibited easily identifiable abnormalities limited to a given locality,[14] and 14 of these had more than a single localized anomaly. The types of abnormalities are summarized in Table 2-1.

The descriptions do not include any abnormalities of the genitourinary system, although there must have been some fetuses with defects of the kidney or ureter, since these are among the more common anomalies in the Spencer collection.

In the group of 560 uterine abortuses classified as normal by Mall, 37 specimens had localized anomalies; [14] of these, 28 had a single defect while 9 possessed multiple faults (Table 2-2).

Relation of Anomalies to Aborton

Before stating conclusions that may be drawn from Tables 2-1 and 2-2, it should be stated that the specimens composing the study group do not

TABLE 2-1
LOCALIZED ANOMALIES IN 38 PATHOLOGIC OVA

Location	Anomaly	No. of ova
Central nervous system	Anencephaly, exencephaly, hydrocephaly, spina bifida, cyclopia	27
Spinal cord	Amyelia	2
Heart	Ectopia	1
Musculoskeletal system	Clubbed foot, clubbed hand, agenesis of radii and thumbs	8
Gastrointestinal tract		1
All systems	Mutiple defects	14
All systems	Single anomaly	24

Data from Mall, F. P., and Meyer, A. W. **Contrib Embryol 12:**198, 1921.

TABLE 2-2
LOCALIZED ANOMALIES IN 37 NORMAL OVA

Location	Anomaly	No. of ova
Central nervous system		20
Musculoskeletal system		5
Gastrointestinal tract	Herniations	3
Genitourinary tract	Ectopia of bladder	1
Double monster		4
Multiple defects		9
Single defect		28

Data from Mall, F. P., and Meyer, A. W. **Contrib Embryol 12:**199, 1921.

represent abortion in the general female population or consecutive cases of abortion in a clinic clientele. The specimens were sent to Mall by physicians who were interested in his work and therefore constitute a group made up chiefly of abnormal or "interesting" fetuses.

Two conclusions stand out. First, there is a very high rate of occurrence of gross anomalies among the abortuses, much higher than the rate of occurrence of the same anomalies among newborn infants. Second, virtually all the fetuses having anomalies in the entire sample of 1000 were aborted in the first half of gestation.

The manner of the collection of specimens increased the bias and decreased the degree of confidence in both the stated conclusions. Still, the great magnitude of the trends deserves notice. On the basis of Mall's observations, it seems likely that proportionately more abnormal than normal fetuses are aborted, since it is the opinion of these investigators that many more abnormal fetuses are lost by abortion than are carried to term as abnormal newborn infants.[14] Both these hypotheses militate against the institution of active treatment of the patient with threatened abortion without obvious maternal cause.

Chromosomal Studies in Abortuses

Chromosomal defects associated with genital abnormalities have been detected in intersex individuals. Other chromosomal aberrations have been detected in aborted fetuses which do not have the stigmata of intersexuality but which have other anomalies, e.g., mongolism. In general, a morphologic defect in the chromosomal karyotype is associated with multiple anatomic anomalies. A number of syndromes of developmental defects, e.g., testicular feminization, are associated with a morphologically normal karyotype but are transmitted through the hereditary mechanism. There are no chromosomal abnormalities identifiable in most cases of single localized anomalies of the genital tract, e.g., bicornuate uterus.

It should be well understood that while chromosomes (genes) may carry traits for developmental anomaly, in many instances, indeed in the overwhelming majority, no morphologic alterations of the chromosomes are seen in the karyotype. An abortus with multiple localized anomalies may have a normal karyotype. Of these individuals we know very little besides empiric data and genetic probabilities.

Chromosomal studies were carried out in specimens of spontaneous abortions and reported in 1965 by Carr.[3] He examined chromosomal preparations cultured from 200 fetuses under 154 days gestational age and found 44 specimens with the chromosomal abnormalities listed in Table 2-3.

The most frequently noted chromosomal anomaly in this study was the X0 pattern (X monosomy), the incidence being 5.5 per cent of the 200 abortuses. Evidence indicates that this rate is some hundreds of times higher than the rate of occurrence of the X0 anomaly in the newborn.

The rate of occurrence of the known syndromes produced by chromosomal trisomies and X chromosomal anomalies is estimated to be about 1 in 245 newborn babies.[15] The discovery by Carr of a rate of 22 per cent chromosomal abnormalities in abortuses represents an incidence of more than 50 times this estimate.

Thiede and Salm studied the chromosomal pattern of 20 aborted fetuses and chorionic vesicles whose tissues grew in culture.[21] Of these, 11 abortuses yielded normal chromosomal patterns, while 9 had an abnormal stem-line or karyotype. Seven of the abortuses were represented by an intact empty sac. All but one of these specimens had abnormal

TABLE 2-3

CHROMOSOMAL ANOMALIES IN 44 ABORTUSES

Anomaly		No. of abortuses
X monosomy (one sex chromosome missing)		11
Triploidy (3 instead of 2 chromosomal sets)		9
Trisomy (one extra chromosome)		22
Trisomy E	7	
Trisomy D	6	
Trisomy G	5	
Trisomy C	2	
Trisomy B	1	
Trisomy A	1	
Tetraploidy		2

Data from Carr, D. **Obstet Gynecol 26:**308, 1965.

chromosomes. A fetus was present in 5 other specimens all but one of which possessed a normal pattern of chromosomes.

Thiede's study included 8 specimens from therapeutic abortion procedures. In all 6 of those done for maternal indications the fetal chromosomes were of normal configuration.

It was considered significant that "there were normal karyotypes in the 6 therapeutic abortions undertaken for maternal indications as well as in the 5 spontaneously aborted normal fetuses (including the tubal pregnancy). Conversely, all the specimens in which there were abnormal karyotypes were associated with some form of fetal and/or placental abnormality." [21]

Many other reports have appeared indicating that a significant proportion of spontaneous abortions is associated with anomalies of the chromosomes in the abortuses.[16, 20] This fact seems particularly impressive in the very young embryos.

Schmid, Jackson *et al.*, and others have reported finding translocation of a chromatin piece in a parent or in the abortus in instances where the mother has had several spontaneous abortions interspersed with successful normal pregnancies.[11, 18] Schmid found a translocation in the G group in a father which was thought to be responsible for abortion of a fetus conceived by him.

Jackson *et al.* studied a family comprising one retarded child, a similarly affected sibling who died in early childhood, two spontaneously aborted embryos not studied cytogenetically, and three normal siblings. One other abortus showed an abnormal karyotype with D-D translocation, as did the living retarded child. This same karyotype was found in the mother, a normal sister, and the maternal grandfather. Thus, the apparent same anomalous karyotype was found in normal individuals, a living but severely abnormal member of the family, and at least one abortus. The chromosomal defect seems to be only partially responsible for the impairments noted.

Summary of Chromosomal Abnormalities in the Fetus

In summarizing information concerning demonstrable chromosomal abnormalities, several generalities may be noted. First, these abnormalities have been identified with a frequency inversely related to the age of individuals studied, the highest proportion of visible defects being in the youngest ones examined and the lowest proportion in living adult human beings. In this connection one would expect that more chromosomal anomalies could be found as younger human beings are investigated, down to and including the ovum and sperm and possibly the embryonic germ cell. The findings of Hertig and Rock, recorded before the advent of scientific study of chromosomes, appears to support this presumption.[10]

Second, the most commonly seen anomalies are those involving sex chromosomes that are more, less, larger, or smaller than the normal ones. More abortuses than newborns are found with an X0 complement, for example, and there are more newborn infants than adults with this complement.

Third, there are many more heritable defects discovered and proved by genetic investigation than there are abnormalities of the karyotypes prepared from tissues of abnormal individuals. To the present time there are relatively few syndromes identifiable in fetus or newborn which are manifestations of morphologic chromosomal defects.

Last, there are contradictions unexplained by present knowledge. It is not known by what mechanism a chromosomal defect produces its somatic manifestation and when a chromosomal defect produces none. Some of the chromosomal defects found in fetuses which have been spontaneously aborted (defects credited with causing the abortion) are also found in living individuals who are the product of term pregnancy. The majority of fetuses aborted spontaneously are anatomically normal, though tissue culture may disclose an abnormal karyotype, e.g., triploidy. The obstetrician usually requests chromosomal study of a congenitally deformed baby in the hope of shedding light upon the cause of the deformity. With few exceptions these studies do not demonstrate chromosomal faults.

Hydatidiform Degeneration and Fetal Anomalies

Hydropic swelling of a few or many chorionic villi along with more or less pronounced degeneration of villous stroma and epithelium have been observed in aborted material for over 125 years.[14] The advanced state of what is apparently the same process results, much less often, in the formation of a "mole" or molar pregnancy, in which the chorionic vesicle is grossly altered by the formation of innumerable watery-looking hydatids attached by stems to the mass. All gradations between the small degree of change or localized hydatidiform degeneration and the generalized conversion of the ovum into a large mass of vesicles have been abundantly described and documented by pictures. Estimates of the frequency of occurrence of hydatidiform mole, the advanced state, vary from 1 in 333 to 1 in 20,000 pregnancies.

Hydatidiform degeneration of chorionic villi in abortuses is found much more frequently, probably proportionately to the diligence with which it is searched for. Mall, for example, found the lesion in 31.5 per cent of 333 pathologic chorionic vesicles of uterine abortuses and in

41.7 per cent of 108 specimens of pathologic tubal pregnancies.[14] The change is undoubtedly more commonly seen in the early months of pregnancy than later. The average age of specimens in the Carnegie collection that showed hydatidiform degeneration was 66 days, or $2\frac{1}{4}$ months.[14] It may be noted, however, that the size of the mass produced by hydropic swelling of the villi is not a reliable guide to fetal age, as it represents degree of involvement rather than length of gestation.

The first signs of hydatidiform degeneration occur in the villous stroma. They are gradual enlargement of the size of the villus, separation of cellular elements, disappearance of villous vessels, supervention of a glassy, bluish transformation of the stroma, and finally replacement of the villous stroma by fluid. All these changes, including the disappearance of villous blood vessels, have been seen by investigators for over a century.[14]

Signs of epithelial proliferation are evident soon after the stromal changes, the degree of change being sometimes so marked as to suggest that it is the primary and not a secondary process. However, some specimens of hydatidiform degeneration show no epithelial proliferation at all, suggesting that the epithelial involvement is not the primary influence in the formation of hydatidiform degeneration.

When the chorionic villi show hydatidiform degeneration, the fetus is usually dead or missing from the amniotic sac. The fetus is smaller than expected from the length of gestation. The state of deterioration or absence of it depends upon how far the disease has progressed before termination by abortion. The occasional coexistence of a living fetus and hydatidiform degeneration of a portion of the placenta might be evidence that fetal death is not the essential cause of the disease process. Hertig and Edmonds commented upon the high rate of occurrence of abnormal fetuses found in association with hydatidiform degeneration of the chorion.[9]

Causes of Hydatidiform Degeneration

Each of the observed pathologic processes has been declared the primary cause of hydatidiform degeneration by one or more investigators. The disappearance of villous blood vessels, the proliferation of the cyto- and syncytiotrophoblast, and the death of the fetus have been said to play a part. Mall thought that "none seems to be better established than . . . endometritis" in causing the change.[14] Of most concern is the possibility of germinal or genetic defect as a cause. The high rate of occurrence of fetal malformation and the higher rate of fetal death (indicating a lethal genetic factor appearing by accident) support a genetic basis. No one yet, to our knowledge, has applied the mathematics of genetics to the question of hydatidiform degeneration. An almost insurmountable obstacle to such a study is the absence of sharp lines of demarcation and definition of which ova are included in the disease group and which ova are normal. The seemingly infinite gradation and degree of hydatidiform change create insoluble problems in classification. One may say, then, that because of the frequency of mild hydatidiform changes and the innumerable gradations, a specific genetic factor is probably not involved.

Summary

Hertig and Edmonds summed up known information and that obtained from a study of their own collection of abortuses by stating that it is appropriate to "regard hydatidiform degeneration more as a physiologic than a purely degenerative process."[9] "The embryo, if one exists in the first place, stops developing at a critical time in the life of the early chorion (about the fifth week of menstrual age). In the absence of any functioning fetal circulation the vascular anlagen of the chorion disappear, and hydatidiform degeneration appears in the very loose stroma of the villi, due in all probability to the continued activity of the trophoblast rather than to any intrinsic degeneration of the stroma."[9] In the case of the clinical hydatidiform mole "this mature manifestation of hydatidiform degeneration varies in no way, except in degree, from that seen frequently in spontaneously aborted pathologic ova which show all gradations in the evolution of the typical lesion."[9]

Chromosomal Studies in Hydatidiform Degeneration

Makino *et al.,* reported chromosomal studies in three specimens of conceptuses showing swollen and edematous chorionic villi "similar to hydatidiform moles."[13] In each case the karyotype prepared from cultured cells showed triploidy (69 XXY). Carr made cytogenetic studies of 13 specimens of spontaneously aborted chorions which exhibited a degree of hydropic swelling of the villi "which were easily visible with the naked eye and indistinguishable, except in degree, from a hydatidiform mole."[4] Carr also reviewed 55 published case reports of chromosomal analyses in cultured cells or in squash preparations from hydatidiform moles. Calling attention to the possible variation in criteria for the diagnosis of hydatidiform mole, he noted that only 7 of the 55 hydatidiform molar specimens showed triploidy (12.7 per cent). Carr stated "there is no doubt that triploidy may occur with or without obvious hydropic changes in the chorionic villi. It now appears that these changes may be found without triploidy. It may be, therefore, that the association of the two conditions is circuitous [sic] and not based on a common etiology."

He speculated that the common factor might be a hormonal imbalance adversely affecting the normal fertilization or cleavage of the egg as well as producing the lesion of the trophoblast.

ANOMALIES IN THE LATE FETUS

Urinary Tract

Potter studied malformations found at autopsy in the late fetus and newborn.[17] Among the anomalies of the urinary tract, she noted *incomplete* and *complete double ureter,* the latter opening into the urinary bladder by two orifices. The incomplete double ureter, or branched ureter, probably caused by premature division of the ureteric bud of the mesonephric duct, is the more frequently encountered variant. The interesting but rare developmental defect of *bilateral renal agenesis* was found to be confined mostly to males.[2, 17] In the few females so affected there were concurrent anomalies of the genital organs, including agenesis of vagina and uterus. The defect in these cases was in the failure of the lower part of the mesonephric duct to grow properly, with the consequent absence of a guide for the müllerian duct and of a source organ for the development of the ureteric bud.

Unilateral renal agenesis was seen in four fetuses in the Spencer collection, whereas two showed bilateral absence of kidneys. Potter's study demonstrated more cases of bilateral than of unilateral absence. In female fetuses with unilateral agenesis of the kidney there was also absence of the müllerian duct on the affected side with unicornuate uterus on the contralateral side.

Genital Tract

In 9000 or more autopsy examinations Potter found a single instance of gonadal agenesis, the baby having the stigmata of *Albright's syndrome* (streak ovaries). This was probably because her examinations did not include a significant proportion of very young fetuses and embryos. In other specimens of fetal ovaries examined she invariably found actively developing follicles containing ova. Furthermore, the follicular activity was evident in all specimens having incomplete or absent müllerian ductal derivatives, thus indicating that absence of müllerian or mesonephric derivatives does not cause absence of gonads or of germ cells in the gonads. This finding is to be expected because of the earlier appearance of the gonads in the time table of development.

Malformations of the internal genital organs are similar to those seen in the adult: absence of part or all of the tubes, uterus, cervix, or vagina,

or arrest of fusion of the müllerian ducts. The anomalous organs differ from those of the adult only in size and secondary sexual maturity. In the male fetus the vasa deferentia, the epididymis, or both may be absent.

Potter found no case of genital malformation characterized by presence of ovotestis.

Associated Malformations

There is a predominance of males among the fetuses with bilateral renal agenesis. Conversely, among babies with anencephaly females predominate in a ratio of approximately 9:1, according to Potter.[35] While Potter found only normal internal organs in all anencephalic babies, one of those in the Spencer collection possessed a bicornuate uterus with rudimentary horn. Absence of at least the lower genital tract (Carnegie No. 6448, Spencer No. A69-22) appears to be the rule in sympodial monsters, the mermaid deformity.[17]

The study of the late fetuses and newborns has reinforced the observations made in other age groups relative to the association of urinary tract and genital tract anomalies. In this group of specimens as well as in those of the younger period of gestation studied by Mall and Meyer, there are more cases of single anomalies than of multiple localized defects. The grouping of such anomalies is well substantiated in the recognition of the several syndromes.

THE SPENCER COLLECTION OF FETUSES

Composition

The Spencer collection of fetuses consists of approximately 1000 specimens consecutively collected and catalogued and another 1000 not catalogued. They were obtained principally from the Admitting Department of Charity Hospital of Louisiana at New Orleans and represent the products of spontaneous abortion delivered either prior to admission to the hospital or shortly thereafter. A few additional fetuses were secured from the wards of Charity Hospital from patients being treated for threatened or inevitable abortion. In a few cases the abortions were induced illegally by nonhospital personnel, but the largest part by far were the result of spontaneous termination of pregnancy. None was obtained by therapeutic abortion.

The patients who aborted were representative of the clientele of the hospital in general. For the most part they were of the lowest socioeconomic level, Negro, and of the young reproductive age group.

Method of Study

Fetuses were examined as soon as possible after collection, usually during the next day. Examinations were carried out before fixation, i.e., in the fresh state. Thus, most specimens were in a near-natural condition when seen. Macerated specimens were examined before fixation also, but the study was, of course, not so satisfactory. Studies were principally gross dissections and examination, where necessary, under the 10- to 20-power binocular dissecting microscope. In the occasional case tissue blocks were secured for histologic sections, but this form of study was not used often. Photographs and drawings recorded abnormal findings, and a few unusual specimens were permanently mounted or placed in formalin.

Purpose

The main purpose of the Spencer study was to elucidate normal and abnormal structure of the gastrointestinal tract and related organs. Inevitably, this involved examination of the external genitalia and the hind end of the body, and scrutiny of this region in turn necessitated examination of the internal genitourinary structures.

The permanent portion of the Spencer collection is essentially records rather than aborted material. It contains results of gross dissections, primarily. It is a study of pathologic changes in fetuses which are due to defective development of the fetus.

The collection is not intended for the study of abortions or causes of abortions except as they are influenced by the anomalous development of the chorion, embryo, or fetus.

Since the specimens were gathered consecutively, the numbers of localized defects give a rough indication of the incidence and the relative incidence of anomalies of the systems.

Observations

The tabulation below and Tables 2-4 and 2-5 list the number of defects found in 430 fetuses which were anomalous. Multiple anomalies occurred in 94 fetuses, single anomalies in 336.

Number of Fetuses Having Localized Anomalies among 1000 Abortuses

Number of fetuses with single anomaly	336
Number of fetuses with multiple anomalies	94

In the genitourinary system the ureter appears to be most often anomalous, although the defects do not interfere with efficient function in

TABLE 2-4

LOCALIZED ANOMALIES IN 430 FETUSES IN THE SPENCER COLLECTION

Type of anomaly	No. of anomalies
Nervous system (hydrocephaly, anencephaly, exencephaly, spina bifida, cyclopia)	6
Muscular system (club foot, etc.)	26
Gastrointestinal system (atresia, malrotation, situs inversus, duplication, imperforate anus)	122
Cardiovascular system	37
Genitourinary system *	62
Omphalomesenteric bands (fetuses 50 mm and over)	137
Adrenal gland, spleen, thymus (agenesis, accessory, ectopia)	179
Miscellaneous, including respiratory	23

* See Table 2-5 for breakdown.

most cases. Defects of the kidneys are frequent and certainly are significant clinically. The Spencer fetuses showed the expected association of
defects of the urinary and the genital systems.

With respect to the internal genital organs, there were relatively few
defective ovaries, only four individual anomalies being found. One would
expect, from the work of other investigators, a larger number of fetuses
exhibiting ovarian agenesis. We could not explain this observation.

TABLE 2-5

ANOMALIES OF THE GENITOURINARY SYSTEM

Type of anomaly	No. of anomalies
Double ureter, branched, uni- or bilateral	15
Hydronephrosis and/or hydroureter	10
Unilateral renal agenesis (all males)	3
Pelvic or "unascended" kidney	7
Horseshoe kidney	3
Bilateral cystic kidneys (both males)	2
Bilateral renal agenesis (both males)	2
Malrotation of kidney (all females)	3
Crossed renal ectopia	1
Urachal cyst	1
Bicornuate uterus (all types)	1
Unicornuate uterus	2
Clitoral hypertrophy	2
Fused labia	1
Absence of external genitalia (sirenomelia)	2
Imperforate urogenital sinus	2
Persistent urogenital sinus	1
Urethra atresia (male)	1
Renal hyperplasia	1
Penile chordee	2

The development of abnormalities of the müllerian system often proved to be triggered by anomalies of the wolffian ductal apparatus, as so often emphasized previously. This causal relation is established by the fact that the appearance of wolffian system antedates that of the müllerian apparatus.

For the specimens in the Spencer collection there were comparatively many localized defects among the fetuses, but the severity of the disorders was certainly no more, and was probably less, than the defects occurring at the time of birth of the defective infant. This suggests that the anomalies did not affect the further development of the gestation. The finding of proportionately more anomalies in aborted fetuses could indicate that anomalies and abortion have common causative factors, rather than that there is a cause and effect relation.

Once again it was noted that anomalies of the organs of the generative system are often coincident with those of the urinary organs.

Finally, it may be noted that since there are so many defects among fetuses aborted early in gestation, the wisdom of treatment to prevent a threatened abortion is questionable.

ILLUSTRATIVE CASE REPORTS

The following case histories illustrate typical anomalies found in the fetus.

Polycystic mesonephros. Carnegie No. 4501; 18 mm, 6½ weeks. Sects. 44-4-4, 44-4-5, 45-2-2. This otherwise normal specimen showed cystic dilation of multiple mesonephric vesicles in the left mesonephros (Fig. 2-1). Only a dozen or so vesicles were involved near the caudal region of the organ. In this locality the dilated vesicles were approximately two to three times the size of the normal-appearing glomeruli. The mesonephric duct may be seen in the near-longitudinal section in *A* and *B*. There were numerous well-developed mesonephric tubules throughout the mesonephros. None of the tubules appeared dilated and neither was the mesonephric duct significantly enlarged. One might consider that there was minimal dilation of the duct in its more caudal portion, but this was not verified at the caudalmost extremity of the duct. The wolffian ducts apparently opened as expected into the urogenital sinus. The thick sections (15 μ) did not allow further analysis of this embryo.

The defect in this case appeared to be a failure of the tubules to connect with either the glomeruli or duct. There was the suggestion of function of the glomeruli inasmuch as they appeared dilated. No fluid was seen, however, on section, an expected finding inasmuch as such fluid would be nonprotein.

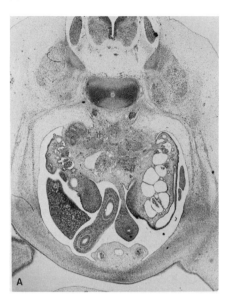

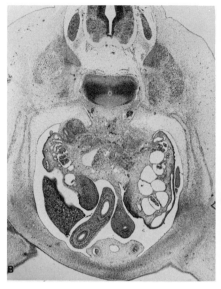

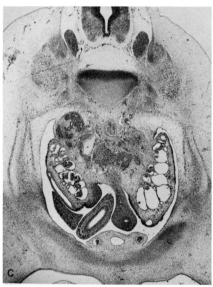

Fig. 2-1. Polycystic disease of left mesonephros (viewer's right). Carnegie No. 4501; A, section 44-4-4; B, section 44-4-5; C, section 45-2-2.

Solitary right ectopic kidney, unicornuate uterus. Spencer No. 1359; 190 mm, 24 weeks. In this specimen (Fig. 2-2) the left kidney and ureter were absent. The right kidney was of approximately normal size for this stage of development but was located at a level just below the bifurcation of the aorta. Aside from the slightly humpbacked contour it was well formed. The ureter was correspondingly shortened.

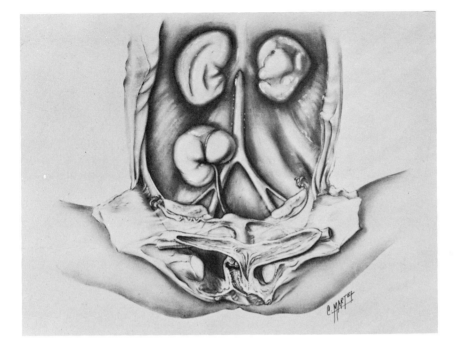

Fig. 2-2. Unicornuate uterus and (solitary right) kidney. Spencer No. 1359. Large adrenal glands are not cap-shaped because neither gland rests on a kidney.

The adrenal glands were in the proper location, near the underside of the diaphragm. Instead of their usual cap-shaped configuration, they were somewhat reniform and flattened. The müllerian system consisted of a normal right fallopian tube, round ligament, and right unicornuate uterus of approximately normal proportions and half of the left fallopian tube. The left müllerian duct was represented by a fallopian tube approximately one-half the expected length. The fimbriated end and cranial one-half of the tube were similar in structure to the counterpart on the right. The caudal half of the left fallopian tube was represented by a thin strand of connective tissue fanning out and ending in the left-sided supports to the uterus. The left round ligament was absent, its location marked by a thin fold of peritoneum extending from the dome of the bladder to the left side of the uterus. Both right and left ovaries appeared completely normal in gross appearance.

When the urinary bladder was opened, the trigone was seen to be partly formed but asymmetrical. The urethral funnel was essentially normal. There was a solitary ureteral orifice on the right normally related to the base of the bladder. There was no orifice in the area where the left ureter should have emptied into the bladder.

The urethra, urethral meatus, vagina, hymen, and vaginal vestibule were normally formed and in their proper relations. The anus was perforate.

Horseshoe kidney, double right ureter, bicornuate uterus, and persistent urogenital sinus. Spencer No. 317; 160 mm, 20 weeks. The kidneys were represented by a single U-shaped mass incorporating about twice the expected amount of kidney parenchyma (Fig. 2-3). The right half of the mass was served by two ureters, separate in their full course. The left side of the kidney was drained by a single ureter. Adrenal glands were essentially normal and in contact with the upper poles of the horseshoe.

The fallopian tubes were normal on both sides with well-formed ostia abdominale. The uterus was of the proper size but its fundus was notched, with a pronounced saddle-shaped depression. Round ligaments were prominent and correctly placed at the sides of the corpus uteri. Ovaries gave the appearance of normal development for this stage.

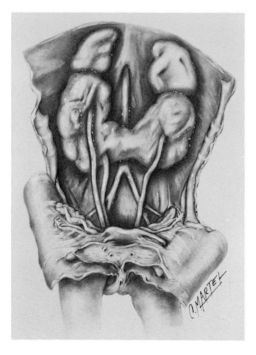

Fig. 2-3. Horseshoe kidney, double right ureter, bicornuate uterus, and persistent urogenital sinus. Spencer No. 317.

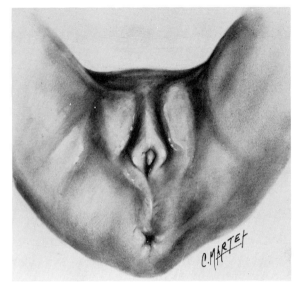

Fig. 2-4. Masculinized external genitalia with fusion of the urethral folds, formation of urogenital sinus just beneath the enlarged clitoris, and labioscrotal folds somewhat ventrally placed. Spencer No. 317.

The topography of the internal surface of the urinary bladder was essentially normal except that at the right corner of the trigone two ureteral orifices could be seen in a somewhat tandem arrangement. The infundibular portion of the bladder led to a short urethra which opened at the base of the clitoris (Fig. 2-4).

The external genitalia were anomalous. There was a single opening at the base of the clitoris and no visible vaginal vestibule. The large labia were somewhat ventral to the point where the vaginal vestibule should have opened. The caudal portions of the labial folds, including the labia minora and majora, were fused in a median raphe, the anal aperture was patent. The appearance of the external genitalia in this case could be said to represent masculinization of the female external genitalia.

Bicornuate uterus with rudimentary horn. Carnegie fetus (unnumbered). This anencephalic, underdeveloped, full-term infant was born with multiple anomalies of the nervous system evident from external examination. The only dissection carried out was that of the internal genitalia (Fig. 2-5). The external genitalia were those of a normal newborn, with well-developed labia, clitoris, vaginal vestibule, and urethral meatus. Both ovaries were grossly normal and properly suspended by the ligaments of the ovaries. Both fallopian tubes were defective in that the ostia abdominales were closed and clubbed, there being no fimbrial cuff. The uterus exhibited the complete bicornuate

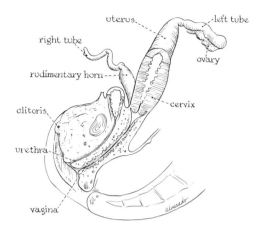

Fig. 2-5. Bicornuate uterus with rudimentary horn and deformed fimbriated ends of tube in anencephalic infant. Unnumbered Carnegie embryo.

configuration with two corpora and one cervix. The left corpus was at least three times as large as the right one. The endometrial cavity was lined by a thin though normal mucosa. The endocervical contours and secretions were normal. The right uterine horn did not contain a recognizable cavity, but instead appeared to be composed of a muscular wall. No communicating channel could be found between the small horn and the cavity of the larger one.

The hymen, vagina, urethra, and urinary bladder were essentially normal.

REFERENCES

1. BRAMBELL, F. W. R. Prenatal mortality in mammals. *Biol Rev 23:*370, 1948.
2. CARPENTIER, P. J., and POTTER, E. L. Nuclear sex and genital malformation in 48 cases of renal agenesis, with especial reference to nonspecific female pseudohermaphroditism. *Am J Obstet Gynecol 78:*235, 1959.
3. CARR, D. Chromosome studies in spontaneous abortions. *Obstet Gynecol 26:*308, 1965.
4. CARR, D. H. Cytogenetics and the pathology of hydatidiform degeneration. *Obstet Gynecol 33:*333, 1969.
5. CORNER, G. W. The problem of embryonic pathology in mammals, with observations upon intrauterine mortality in the pig. *Am J Anat 31:*523, 1923.
6. CORNER, G. W., and BARTELMEZ, G. W. Early abnormal embryos of the Rhesus monkey. *Contrib Embryol 35:*1, 1954.
7. FRAZER, J. F. D. Foetal death in the rat. *J Embryol Exp Morphol 3:*13, 1955.
8. HERTIG, A. T., ROCK, J., and ADAMS, E. C. A description of 34 human ova within the first 17 days of development. *Am J Anat 98:*435, 451, 457, 1956.
9. HERTIG, A. T., and EDMONDS, H. W. Genesis of hydatidiform mole. *Arch Pathol 30:*260, 287, 289, 290, 1940.

10. HERTIG, A. T., ROCK, J., ADAMS, E. C., and MENKIN, M. C. Thirty-four fertilized human ova, good, bad and indifferent, recovered from 210 women of known fertility. *Pediatrics 23*:202, 1959.

11. JACKSON, P., DUPONT, A., and MIKKELSEN, M. Translocation in the 13–15 group as a cause of partial trisomy and spontaneous abortion in the same family. *Lancet 2*:584, 1963.

12. LEWIS, W. N., and HARTMAN, C. G. Tubal ova of the Rhesus monkey. *Contrib Embryol 29*:15, 1941.

13. MAKINO, S., SASAKI, M. S., and FUKUSCHIMA, T. Triploid chromosomal constitution in human chorionic lesions. *Lancet 2*:1273, 1964.

14. MALL, F. P., and MEYER, A. W. Studies on abortuses: A survey of pathologic ova in the Carnegie embryological collection. *Contrib Embryol 12*:43, 44. 185, 194, 198, 199, 203, 210, 215, 221, 225, 1921.

15. MARDEN, P. M., SMITH, D. W., and McDONALD, M. J. Congenital anomalies in the newborn infant, including minor variations. *J Pediatr 64*:357, 1964.

16. MOTOMICHI, S., SAJIRO, M., JUN-ICHI, M., TATSURO, I., and HACHIRO, S. A chromosome survey of induced abortuses in a Japanese population. *Chromosoma (Berl) 20*:267, 1967.

17. POTTER, E. L. *Pathology of the Fetus and the Newborn.* Chicago, Year Book, pp. 385, 417, 1952.

18. SCHMID, W. A familial chromosome abnormality associated with repeated abortions. Cytogenetics *1*:199, 1962.

19. SCHULTZ, A. H. Sex incidence in abortions. In Mall and Meyer, R., *op. cit.,* pp. 177, 181.

20. SMITH, M., MACNAB, J., and FERGUSON-SMITH, M. A. Cell culture techniques for cytogenetic investigation of human aborted material. *Obstet Gynecol 33*:313, 1969.

21. THIEDE, H. A., and SALM, S. Chromosome studies of human spontaneous abortions. *Am J Obstet Gynecol 90*:205, 213, 1964.

Chapter Three

Anomalies in the Infant

Rowena Spencer

Any derangement of the structure of the genital tract in infancy must be regarded as significant, because of the possibilities of associated anomalies, future marital or obstetric difficulties, or erroneous sex assignment.

While it would be inappropriate in the newborn period to attempt to determine the minute anatomic details of internal viscera which are not expected to function for at least another decade, the external genitalia can and should be carefully examined. If no external anomalies are found, it will then remain for gynecologic or obstetric evaluation in adolescent or adult life to detect developmental anomalies of the internal genitalia. However, any time urinary tract malformations are diagnosed during childhood, the genitalia should be reexamined for anomalies which might have been overlooked previously.

MALFORMATIONS OF THE EXTERNAL GENITALIA AND HIND END OF THE BODY

Abnormalities of the external genitalia should be diagnosed on the routine physical examination in the newborn period. While the local anomaly may not of itself be significant, it indicates the possibility of anomalies in other organs. Campbell [4] states that there are anomalies of the upper tract in one-third of the patients with genital malformations and that two-thirds of the females who have upper tract abnormalities also have anomalies of the genitalia.

Examination of the external genitalia in the newborn period should confirm the normal gross anatomy, not only of the labia majora and minora, but also of the mons veneris and the underlying symphysis pubis; not only of the clitoris and the edematous and protruding hymen, but also of the urethra lying in the angle between the two. Even the umbilicus deserves attention here, not only its location but also its content. Absence of the infraumbilical abdominal wall (juxtaposition of the umbilicus and the external genitalia) and absence of the umbilical artery are both associated with a high incidence of anomalies, particularly in the urogenital system.

The examination should include separation of the labia, which are swollen and edematous in response to the maternal hormones, and confirmation of the patency of the hymen and the vagina, either indirectly, by noting the copious, tenacious secretions of the endocervical glands, or directly by inserting a sterile blunt probe if necessary. Rectal examination, even with the smallest of adult digits, produces painful superficial lacerations in the anal canal and so rarely yields any useful information that it is not recommended as part of the routine examination in normal infants. It is enough simply to ascertain (with a thermometer) that the anus is patent and in its normal location within, not anterior to, the external anal sphincter. The coccyx and sacrum should be palpated and this area carefully inspected for bony defects and congenital dermal sinuses.

Since the internal genital organs (gonads and müllerian apparatus) develop independently of one another, anomalies in each of these structures must be considered in separate categories. However, the development of the external organs of the genital system (genital tubercle, labioscrotal folds, and cloacal membrane) is so intimately interrelated that isolated anomalies are rare, and abnormalities of the external genitalia are considered as one single group.

Most abnormalities of the external genitalia fall into the classification of "malformations of the hind end of the body" in which there is a high incidence of anomalies in the structures derived from all three germ layers in this region: the cloaca, cloacal membrane, external genitalia, anterior abdominal wall, and lower vertebral column and spinal cord. These malformations fall into four groups: (1) agenesis, (2) embryonic fissure, (3) embryonic arrest or distortion, and (4) duplication.

Agenesis

Malformations resulting from agenesis vary in extent from absence of the entire hind end of the body, through absence of all the external genitalia, to isolated absence of the phallus.

Sympodia

Absence of the entire hind end of the body results in the condition known as *sympodia* (sirenomelia, sympus apus, or mermaid), which is characterized by fusion of the two lower extremities into one limb with the conjoined foot either resembling the flippers of a seal or missing altogether. Whether the specific embryologic defect be aplasia, atrophy, or degeneration, the effect is that of early embryonic destruction of the entire "hind end of the body," including the caudal (posterolateral) portion of the lower extremities, the entire perineum and underlying cloaca, and frequently the coccyx and sacrum (Fig. 3-1). During the subsequent healing of this extensive but localized defect, the caudal aspects of the lower extremities become fused together in the midline, the resulting external rotation so severe that the patella may come to occupy the posterior aspect of the conjoined limb.

Since the perineum is obliterated, there are no urinary, genital, or anal orifices and no external genitalia, although a structure resembling a tail or a phallus may occasionally be found. Destruction of the caudal extent of the cloaca prevents the formation of the urinary tract. If there is no cloaca into which the mesonephric ducts empty, the lower ends of these ducts do not develop normally, so that there may be no metanephric ducts. If the metanephric ducts are absent, there can be no metanephros, since the ducts induce the formation of the kidney from the nephrogenic blastema. There is frequently no urinary tract at all in the sympodial fetus, but occasionally small cystic kidneys or remnants of mesonephros are found in the retroperitoneal tissue.

Absence of the cloacal membrane and the lowest portion of the cloaca results in imperforate anus and absence of the rectum. The caudal extent of the colon ends blindly in the lower abdomen.

Since there is no urogenital sinus with which the müllerian ducts can communicate, there is no perineal orifice for the female genital tract. This disturbance in the development of the lower ends of the müllerian system usually prevents the two lateral ducts from fusing properly in midline, resulting in two widely separated unicornuate uteri. The gonads and the fallopian tubes or the epididymi are usually normal, but the lower ends of the reproductive tracts disappear in the depths of the abnormal pelvis.

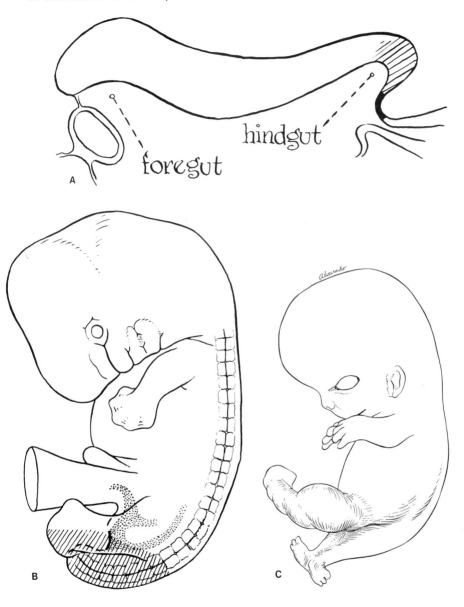

Fig. 3-1. Artist's concept of the embryology of sympodia in the 2-, 12-, and 30-mm embryo (*A, B,* and *C,* respectively). Area of destruction is cross-hatched in *A* and *B*. In *B,* allantois-hindgut-cloaca is stippled, and cloacal membrane is represented by heavy black line beneath tailfold.

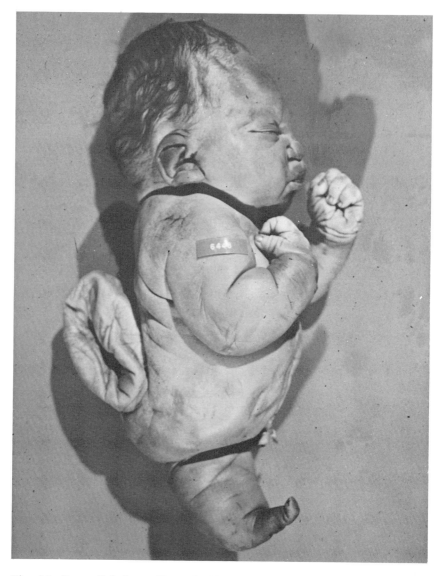

Fig. 3-2. Sympodial fetus. Carnegie No. 6448. Note large myelomeningocele
and absence of external genitalia.

A single midline umbilical artery is the hallmark of the typical mermaid. Embryonic destruction (or absence) of most of the tissue which
normally develops between these two vessels permits the formation of
one, not two, umbilical arteries. In spite of the abnormally high origin
of this single umbilical artery from the abdominal aorta, it is not an
omphalomesenteric artery as has been suggested,[43] for it follows an extra-
peritoneal course. The omphalomesenteric vessels traverse the free peritoneal cavity.

The profound external rotation of the lower extremities that accompanies the fusion of the two femurs into one bone and the two acetabula
into one joint results in a severe lordosis and extreme distortion of the
pelvis. The iliac bones may be fused posteriorly if the sacrum is absent
and are directed more laterally and inferiorly than normal. The ischial
spines and tuberosities are often joined in the posterior midline, and the
two pubic bones fuse, not only in the area of the symphysis, but also
along the inferior rami. This produces a shallow, narrow pelvic space
directed anteriorly.

Despite the severity of the malformation in these patients, abnormalities are rare in areas other than the hind end of the body, suggesting
that this is indeed a localized defect.

The two mermaid fetuses in this series were both females, in contrast
to the high incidence of males usually reported with this anomaly.

Sympodia. Carnegie No. 6448. A 6-pound fetus with sirenomelia and a
  lumbar myelomeningocele was normal above the umbilicus (Fig. 3-2).
  The single tapered lower extremity curved anteriorly. There were no
  external genitalia and no kidneys, ureters, or bladder. The ovaries
  and fallopian tubes were normal in configuration but close together
  in the midline (Fig. 3-3). The unicornuate uterus on each side extended directly inferiorly and disappeared in the abdominal wall. A
  heavy fibrous band connected the internal genitalia across the prominent single umbilical artery.

Sympodia. A69-22. This full-term female sympodial fetus had no external
  genitalia (Fig. 3-4). The ovaries and fallopian tubes were normal. The
  lower ends of the tubes disappeared in the retroperitoneal space on
  either side of the single umbilical artery (Fig. 3-5). Two small cystic
  kidneys on the left side shared a single Y-shaped ureter, and there
  was no external orifice for the bladder, which contained a few drops
  of fluid and filled the entire pelvis. An additional abnormality in this
  fetus was a small accessory diaphragm in the right hemithorax.

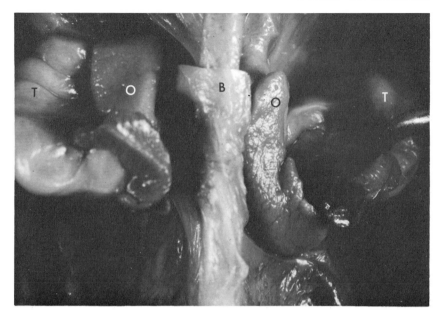

Fig. 3-3. Internal genitalia of female sympodial fetus. Carnegie No. 6448. Note ovaries (O), fallopian tubes (T), and band of fibrous tissue (B) connecting lower ends of tubes across prominent single umbilical artery.

Absence of the External Genitalia

Absence may result in a smooth unblemished perineum or in absence of the perineum with a web between the partially fused thighs. The external orifices of the urogenital and gastrointestinal tracts are absent, an abnormality obviously incompatible with extrauterine life. The duration of fetal life may vary inversely with renal function: the anuric (anephric) infant may reach full term, but the fetus with kidneys which do produce urine may acquire a bladder so distended that it literally fills the abdomen and interferes with the development of the other viscera.

Absence of the perineum with other anomalies. CH50-438608. This premature infant lived only 1 hour. Autopsy revealed gastroschisis; absense of the vulva, vagina, anus, gallbladder, right kidney, and lungs; hypoplasia of the adrenals; and multiple cardiac defects. There was no description of the general appearance of the infant (or the perineum) before or after death, nor were the uterus, tubes, or ovaries mentioned.

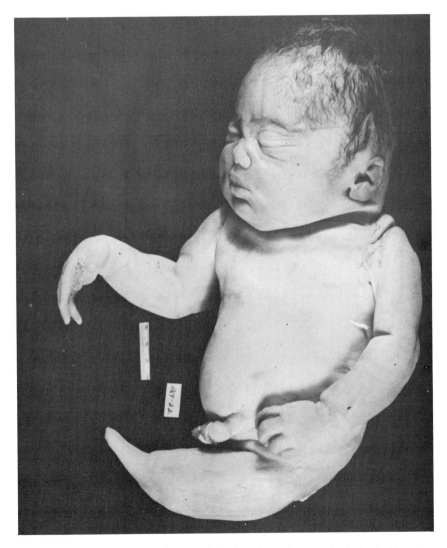

Fig. 3-4. Sympodial fetus with Potter's facies of renal agenesis. A69-22. (Courtesy of Dr. John H. Dent, Jr., New Orleans.)

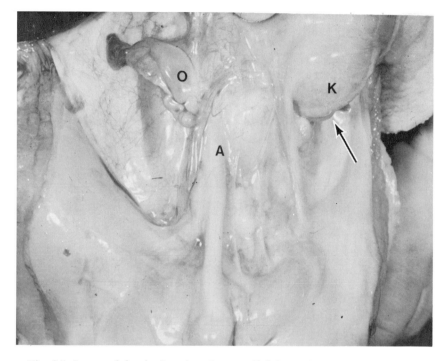

Fig. 3-5. Lower abdominal cavity of sympodial fetus. A69-22. Note absence of uterus. Normal right tube and ovary (*O*) are near single midline umbilical artery (*A*). Left tube (*arrow*) is just visible beneath cystic left kidney (*K*).

Isolated Absence of the Phallus

This is a rare condition; the incidence said to be similar in the two sexes.[4] Neither absence nor duplication of the phallus (see below) has the same significance in the female as in the male, since the female without a clitoris does not necessarily have any associated anomaly of the urethra or difficulties with procreation.

The only apparent instances of absence of the clitoris among our patients occurred in those with exstrophy of the bladder in whom the small, bifid, laterally displaced clitoris probably escaped recognition.

Embryonic Fissure

Abnormalities resulting from an anomalous fissure through the infra-umbilical abdominal wall include exstrophy of the cloaca, exstrophy of the bladder, and epispadias.[11, 27, 39, 46]

In the human embryo of about 2 weeks (fertilization age) the fetal body is a thin disc of cells lying between the amniotic cavity above and

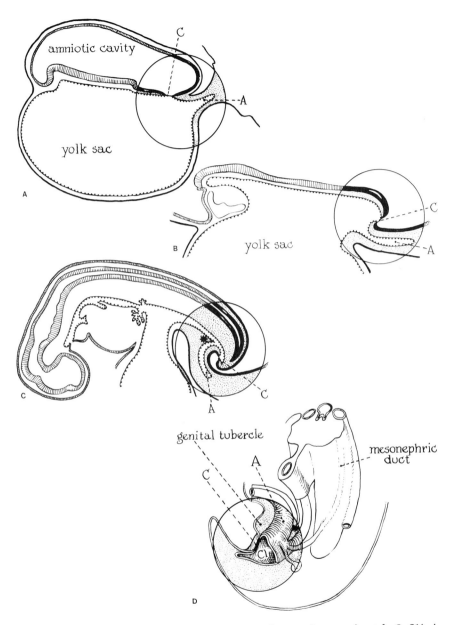

Fig. 3-6. Diagrammatic sections of human embryos of approximately 2, 2½, 4, and 5 weeks. Area of interest is circled. *A* indicates allantois; *C*, cloacal membrane; *Cl*, cloaca. Ectoderm is shown by heavy black line; endoderm by beaded line; mesoderm by stippled area. Urorectal fold is indicated by asterisk in *C* and *D*. (From Spencer, R. *Surgery* 57:751, 1965.)

the yolk sac below (Fig. 3-6*A*). Posterior to the embryonic disc, the cloa-cal membrane is represented by a linear area of fusion of the amniotic ectoderm with the yolk sac endoderm. The allantois extends into the body stalk from that portion of the yolk sac which later becomes the cloaca.

During the third week, longitudinal growth of the embryo results in the formation of both head- and tailfolds (Fig. 3-6*B*), so that (1) a small portion of the yolk sac is incorporated into each end of the body to form the foregut and the hindgut, and (2) the cloacal membrane is brought to lie on the ventral aspect of the body, extending to or onto the body stalk. At this time there is no infraumbilical abdominal wall.

As the body walls continue to close in ventrally, more of the yolk sac is included within the body, and the communication between the yolk sac and the midgut area is progressively constricted (Fig. 3-6*C*). At the same time, mesoderm migrating from the primitive streak of the tailfold grows between the ectoderm and the endoderm caudal to the body stalk to establish the beginning of a lower abdominal wall. This process re-duces the anatomic extent of the cloacal membrane to an area later to become the perineum. Further accumulations of mesoderm form the genital tubercle, the labioscrotal folds, and the anal tubercles anterior, lateral, and posterior to the cloacal membrane.

The mesonephric ducts, from which the metanephric ducts (ureters) later branch, open into the anterolateral walls of the cloaca at about 4 weeks. The area into which they open will become the bladder after the urorectal fold grows down to the perineum to divide the cloaca into rectum and urogenital sinus (Fig. 3-6*D*). The urorectal fold reaches the perineum at about 7 weeks, so that perforation of the cloacal membrane shortly thereafter produces two orifices, anal and urogenital. The mül-lerian ducts reach the urogenital sinus at about 9 weeks, and the uro-genital system is subsequently further modified depending upon the sex of the embryo.

The cloacal membrane constitutes a vulnerable area on the infraum-bilical abdominal wall. Should the membrane perforate prematurely in its primitive location, or should the ingrowing mesoderm fail to reduce its primitive extent, the resulting fissure through the abdominal wall will open into the anterior wall of the cloaca in the area destined to become the urinary bladder. The timing of the perforation and the sub-sequent interference with development in the immediate vicinity deter-mines the extent of the resulting defect—exstrophy of the cloaca, ex-strophy of the bladder, or simply epispadias ("exstrophy of the urethra").

Exstrophy of the Cloaca

This condition (Fig. 3-7) results from a perforation through the anterior abdominal wall into the primitive unpartitioned cloaca, with subsequent failure of the urorectal fold to separate the rectum from the bladder–urogenital sinus area.[37] This vesicoabdominal fissure produces exstrophy of a wide expanse of viscera consisting of two lateral areas of bladder separated by a central portion of bowel. The exposed bowel must be ileocecal region, as both ileal and colonic mucosa and the orifice of the appendix are found in the exstrophy.

The abnormal opening into the cloaca is very short in actual measurement at the time it occurs, but very long in terms of length of bowel destined to have formed from this portion of the primitive gut. The interference with normal longitudinal growth significantly shortens the

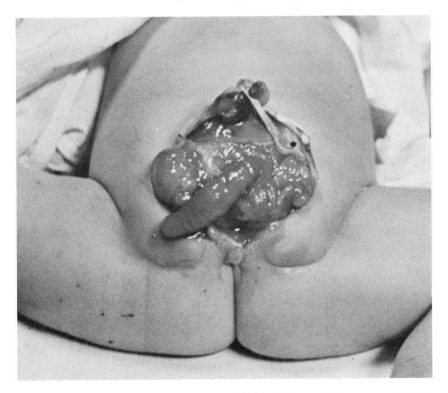

Fig. 3-7. Exstrophy of the cloaca. CH56-216092. Note widely separated labia majora lateral to two halves of clitoris, each with its labium minus. Prolapsed ileum protrudes between two halves of exstrophic bladder.

large bowel and, occasionally, the ileum. The exposed cecum and a short blind tube of colon which develops distal to the exstrophy constitute the entire large intestine.

Other malformations of the urogenital apparatus (phallus, labioscrotal folds, and orifices of the ureters, vagina, and vas deferens) are secondary to the abnormal division of the urogenital sinus into two lateral halves. The fissure through the lower abdominal wall prevents the two pubic bones from meeting in the midline to form a symphysis. This results in diastasis of the lower portions of the rectus muscles, which may be a factor in the development of the omphalocele often associated with exstrophy of the cloaca.

The most striking feature of the typical case of exstrophy of the cloaca is a large area of exposed mucosa on the lower abdominal wall, usually surmounted by an omphalocele. The midportion of the exstrophy consists of intestinal mucosa surrounding one to four identifiable orifices. Through the most superior orifice the terminal ileum is often prolapsed, while the most inferior one leads into a short blind colon. Either one or two appendices may open on the lateral aspects of the exstrophied intestine or the appendix may be absent. The anus is invariably imperforate, although occasionally a proctodeal dimple is described.

On each side of the exposed bowel is an area of exstrophied bladder mucosa. The two portions of the bladder are usually entirely separated by bowel but may be continuous above or below it or may completely encircle it. The ureteral orifices and occasionally the openings of the vasa deferentia or the vaginas may be found on the bladder mucosa. The testes are usually undescended and the external genitalia are either absent or are abnormally formed, the phallus being represented by a short broad midline structure with epispadias or by two widely separated diminutive papillae. The lower portions of the labia majora or the empty scrotal folds usually meet in the midline below the area of the exstrophy but may be so widely separated as to appear to be on the upper thighs.

There is always diastasis pubis, the two ends of the pubis being directed anteriorly in the area below the exstrophy. Abnormalities of the vertebral column, ranging from simple hemivertebrae through spina bifida to myelomeningocele, occur frequently and are usually associated with some degree of clubfoot.

Operation or autopsy reveals absence of a large part of the colon. There may be no identifiable bowel distal to the exstrophy, but usually a short tube of colon opens off the lower portion of the exstrophy and ends blindly in front of the sacrum. Rotation of the midgut is frequently imperfect, and the inferior mesenteric artery is usually missing, since the bowel normally supplied by this vessel is absent.

In females the two halves of the müllerian apparatus fail to fuse in the midline, and two vaginas may connect with the ureters or with the surface of the bladder. Similarly, in the male the vasa deferentia may empty into the ureters or to the surface of the bladder. Conversely, the ureters may drain into the vaginas or vasa deferentia. Absence of one umbilical artery may be accompanied by agenesis or abnormality of the ipsilateral kidney and/or gonad. Other anomalies of the upper urinary tract are common, including cystic kidney, pelvic kidney, hydronephrosis, hydroureter, and duplication or atresia of the ureter.

Four newborn infants at Charity Hospital were diagnosed as having typical exstrophy of the cloaca. Three (CH59-315710, CH56-216092, and CH53-116891) had repair of the coexisting omphalocele and construction of an ileostomy and died of pulmonary complications; two had troublesome fluid loss from the ileostomy. The fourth infant (CH50-400805) had repair of the omphalocele only and died of persistent vomiting; autopsy was not done.

Exstrophy of the cloaca. CH67-170850. This infant was noted at birth to have severe undiagnosed malformations of the abdominal wall and perineum (Fig. 3-8). In spite of inability to identify the external genitalia, the infant was said to be a male. After two attempts at closure, the small omphalocele was allowed to epithelize spontaneously. The exstrophy of the bladder was recognized and when the upper urinary tract could not be visualized by excretory or retrograde urography,

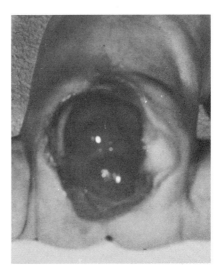

Fig. 3-8. Exstrophy of the cloaca with a large hernia into exstrophied bowel. CH67-170850.

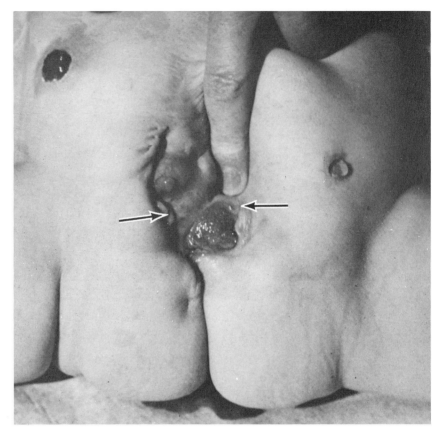

Fig. 3-9. Exstrophy of the cloaca after excision of exstrophied bowel and ap–
proximation of two halves of bladder in the midline. CH67-170850. Note left
cutaneous ureterostomy and right lower quadrant colostomy. *Arrows* indicate
two halves of clitoris.

the infant was thought to be too hopelessly deformed to survive and
so was sent home to die.

At 3½ weeks she weighed 5 lb, 11 oz (birth weight had been 6 lb,
8 oz) and was severely dehydrated and malnourished. Exposed bowel
and bladder mucosa were typical of exstrophy of the cloaca. The external genitalia were bifid and widely separated but typically female
(Fig. 3-9). There was imperforate anus but no abnormality of the
vertebral column, the lower extremities, or the upper half of the body
(except a bifid right thumb).

At operation, the infant was found to have exstrophy of the cloaca atypical only in that the colon was of normal length. (There was only one appendix.) The right kidney and ureter were normal, but the left kidney was small and the ureter obstructed at the ureterovesical junction. The two unicornuate uteri were separated by the exstrophied bowel and the two hemivaginas opened onto the lower portions of the exstrophied bladder mucosa.

A left ureterostomy and colostomy were done and the exstrophy of the bowel excised; the abdomen was closed by bringing together the two halves of the bladder (Fig. 3-9). Subsequent growth and development were normal, and at age 2 years the bladder was excised, urinary diversion accomplished through an isolated loop of colon, and the vagina opened beneath the approximated halves of the clitoris.

Exstrophy of the Bladder

This anomaly has its origin before the fifth week of embryonic life, when the genital tubercle makes its appearance as a conical thickening of the mesoderm between the anterior extent of the cloacal membrane and the inferior margin of the body stalk. Prior to this time, there is no infraumbilical abdominal wall, the cloacal membrane extending up to (or onto) the lowermost portion of the body stalk (Fig. 3-6).

A disturbance in the development of this area—be it rupture of the cloacal membrane in its primitive position, posterior displacement of the genital tubercle,[35] or failure of the mesodermal elements to reach the infraumbilical abdominal wall—results in a fissure through the anterior abdominal wall and into the cloaca. Should the urorectal fold normally partition the cloaca into rectum and bladder either before or after the perforation of the cloacal membrane, the defect may result in exstrophy of the bladder with an intact colon and rectum (Fig. 3-10). Not uncommonly, local disturbance in the cloacal membrane or in the surrounding mesoderm also produces an imperforate anus. Exstrophy of the bladder with imperforate anus and rectovesical fistula is differentiated from atypical exstrophy of the cloaca by the location of the fistula at the base of the bladder (or the urethra) in the former condition and on the posterior wall of the bladder in the latter. In addition, the colon is usually of normal length in exstrophy of the bladder but rarely so in exstrophy of the cloaca. Varying degrees of anomalies in the genital, urinary, alimentary, skeletal, and nervous systems which occur with exstrophy of the cloaca also accompany exstrophy of the bladder.

In typical exstrophy of the bladder, the umbilical cord is located at the superior border of the exstrophic bladder mucosa. Subsequent fibrosis around the periphery of the exstrophy may obliterate the umbilical scar. The entire infraumbilical abdominal wall is split; there is no mons veneris or underlying symphysis pubis. Instead, there is diastasis pubis with the everted bladder mucosa forming a protruding erythematous mass in the lower midline of the abdominal wall. Examination of the abnormal genitalia reveals the upper portions of the labia to be widely separated, with a diminutive half of a clitoris surmounting each labium minus, one on each side of the exstrophic bladder mucosa. (The male patient will usually have epispadias instead of a bifid phallus, but this is rare in females.) The vaginal orifice is usually normal but may not be recognized on casual inspection.

There were 13 cases of exstrophy of the bladder in females at Charity Hospital. (There were 39 males.) Of the 13 females, 4 were admitted as newborns, 3 were 1½–5 months old, and 6 were 4–34 years of age at the time of the first admission. Two newborns (CH55-19544 and CH65-99089, Fig. 3-11) had intraabdominal bladders with a bifid clitoris, separation of the anterior portions of the labia, diastasis pubis, and incontinence (female epispadias); all other cases apparently had typical exstrophy.

In only 3 patients (all newborn) was there an adequate description of the external genitalia. All had bifid clitoris with separation of the labia anteriorly but with a normal vaginal orifice. The fourth patient admitted as a newborn was subjected to uretero-sigmoidostomy at age 6 months, when the uterus and vagina were not identified. Six years later, when an ileal loop was constructed for urinary diversion, the surgeon described the tubes and ovaries as being normal and the uterus as rudimentary.

Only 3 patients were noted to have congenital anomalies other than those of the hind end of the body: a newborn had dextrocardia (which was asymptomatic at 16 years of age), another had gastroschisis, and a 4-year-old had a congenital heart defect. In this patient, an omphalocele and clubfeet were considered to have resulted from the same disturbance in development that produced the exstrophy.

Exstrophy of the bladder. CH65-106363. The patient was sent to Charity Hospital on the day of birth because of uncertainty about sex assignment and question about the diagnosis of the lower abdominal wall defect (Fig. 3-10). She was found to have a typical exstrophy of the bladder with a bifid clitoris but a normal vaginal orifice. Reconstructive surgery was deferred until the age of 2 years, since the upper urinary tract was normal.

Lesser degrees of abdominal fissure consist of either bifid clitoris or epispadias, with the fissure occasionally extending into the bladder neck, usually with an accompanying diastasis pubis.

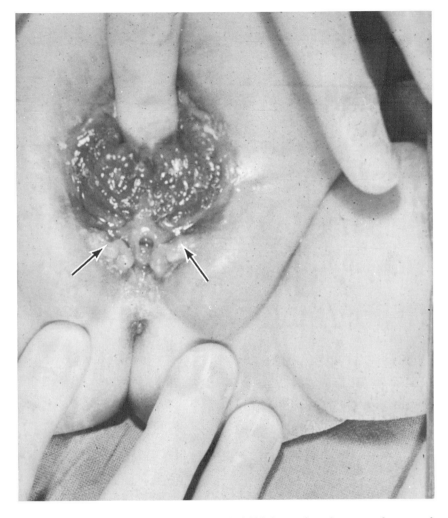

Fig. 3-10. Exstrophy of the bladder with bifid but otherwise normal external genitalia. CH65-106363. Vaginal orifice is between two halves of clitoris (*arrows*).

Bifid clitoris with diastasis pubis (female epispadias). CH65-99098. In this infant, born with gastroschisis, almost the entire gastrointestinal tract had herniated through a small defect at the base of the umbilical cord (Fig. 3-11). In addition, there was absence of the infraumbilical abdominal wall, with the edge of the umbilical defect only 1 cm or so above the genitalia, but there was no exstrophy of the bladder. The clitoris was bifid, the upper portions of the labia were widely sepa-

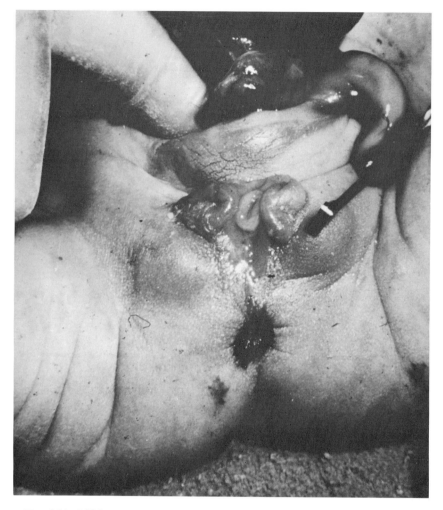

Fig. 3-11. Bifid external genitalia associated with absence of infraumbilical abdominal wall and gastroschisis. CH65-99098. Edematous hymen protrudes between widely separated labia minora.

rated, and there was an associated diastasis pubis. The vaginal and anal orifices were normal.

At operation, it was possible to cover most of the bowel with mobilized abdominal skin; the remainder of the bowel was covered with Marlex. Granulation tissue slowly separated the Marlex from the bowel and the defect eventually epithelized. The huge abdominal hernia was closed at the age of 2 years. At this time it was apparent that the bladder neck was involved in the fissure through the abdominal wall, since the child was incontinent of urine.

Embryonic Arrest or Distortion

Anorectal and Perineal Anomalies

Among the more frequent abnormalities of the external genitalia are those associated with anorectal anomalies ("imperforate anus"). That these are indeed malformations of the hind end of the body and not just localized abnormalities of the anus is indicated by a high incidence of associated anomalies in the lower vertebral column and the upper urinary tract.

The pathologic embryology responsible for the formation of these anorectal malformations involves the tailgut and the caudal portion of the primitive cloaca, the cloacal membrane itself, and the mesoderm which enters into the formation of the perineum.

In a 2-week human embryo, the cloacal membrane is an area of fusion of the yolk sac endoderm with the amniotic ectoderm posterior to the caudal extent of the embryonic disc (Fig. 3-6*A*). Thus at this very early stage of development, the future cloacal lumen is already in contact with the cloacal membrane, and any theory of the etiology of imperforate anus must include a logical explanation for the disruption of this primitive cloaca–cloacal membrane relation.

Formation of the tailfold brings the cloacal membrane to lie on the ventral aspect of the body, extending up to the body stalk (Fig. 3-6*B*). Subsequent ingrowth of mesoderm between the body stalk and the cloacal membrane establishes the beginning of an infraumbilical abdominal wall, forms the genital tubercle, and limits the cloacal membrane to the area of the perineum.

Shortly after the formation of the tail, the tailgut makes its appearance as a tubular extension of the posterior-inferior portion of the cloaca (Fig. 3-6*D*). Almost as soon as it is formed, the tailgut begins to disintegrate, and the area of the cloaca from which it arose closes over. The caudal portion of the cloaca (the rectal anlage) remains intact and the cloacal membrane is undisturbed.

The cloaca is then partitioned into two chambers by the urorectal fold (Fig. 3-6*D*), a saddle-shaped wedge of mesoderm which grows caudally in the angle between the allantois and the hindgut, the two caudal extremities of the fold progressing toward the midline while the apex descends toward the perineum.

Three mesodermal accumulations participate in the formation of the mesenchymal structures of the perineum: (1) the urorectal fold just de-

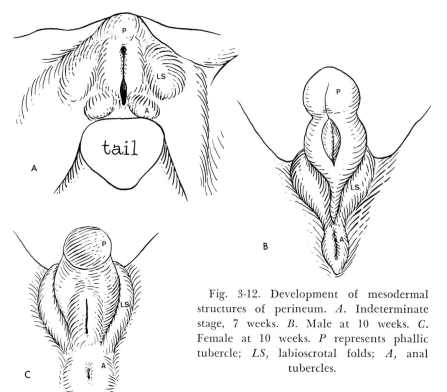

Fig. 3-12. Development of mesodermal structures of perineum. *A.* Indeterminate stage, 7 weeks. *B.* Male at 10 weeks. *C.* Female at 10 weeks. *P* represents phallic tubercle; *LS,* labioscrotal folds; *A,* anal tubercles.

scribed; (2) the anal tubercles, which appear just beneath the tailfold and grow anteriorly along the posterolateral aspects of the cloacal membrane; and (3) the labioscrotal folds, which similarly buttress the anterolateral portions of the cloacal membrane (Fig. 3-12). The urorectal fold from above, the anal tubercles from behind, and the labioscrotal folds from in front, all arrive at the midpoint of the perineum at about the same time, closing the perineum between the anal and urogenital membranes, forming the perineal body, and deepening the anal canal and the urogenital groove. The urogenital membrane perforates almost as soon as it is partitioned from the cloacal membrane, and the anal membrane breaks down a short time later.

Continued fusion of the urethral folds anteriorly from the midpoint of the perineum closes the urogenital groove to form the male urethra, and the coalescence of the mesoderm of the labioscrotal folds across the midline forms the scrotum. In the female, the junction of the müllerian ducts with the urogenital sinus at the site of the müllerian tubercle is some considerable distance from the perineum. The urogenital sinus caudal to the müllerian tubercle subsequently widens in an antero-posterior direction and becomes relatively more shallow. Thus the uro-genital groove and the distal urogenital sinus are converted into the vaginal vestibule, and the vaginal and urethral orifices are brought down closer to the perineum.

True imperforate anus. This is a rare anomaly consisting of a fibrous or membranous atresia at the mucocutaneous junction of the anus (Fig. 3-13E). The perineum appears normal until the anal canal is exposed, and there is no associated fistula to the urogenital system. This anomaly is easily explained by the absence of perforation of the anal membrane after normal development of the rectum and the perineum.

Most other anorectal anomalies are probably related to excessive re-sorption of the tailgut, resulting in disintegration of the endodermal lining of the anal membrane and destruction of a variable portion of the rectal anlage.[6,7] Subsequent ingrowth of mesoderm obliterates the thin area previously occupied by the anal membrane and prevents its normal perforation. The communication between the remaining rectal anlage and the cloaca will persist as a rectourogenital fistula (Fig. 3-13A).

Rectoperineal fistula. The most superficial of these abnormalities prob-ably results from destruction of only the endodermal lining of most of the anal membrane. The remaining small "anal" orifice is displaced anteriorly as a rectoperineal fistula, but the underlying rectum is usually normal (Figs. 3-13F and 3-14). After the endodermal lining of the anal membrane disappears, fusion of the anal tubercles over the normal loca-tion of the anal orifice frequently produces a broad thick midline raphe. In most of these patients, as well as those with more extensive defects, foreshortening of the perineum and/or absence of the perineal body are evidence of abnormal development of both mesodermal and endodermal elements of the perineum.

Recto–fossa navicularis and rectovaginal fistulae. More extensive de-struction of the cloaca, involving not only the anal membrane but also the lower portion of the rectal anlage, would result in absence of the anal orifice and of the lower rectum. In these cases there is usually a fistula from the remaining (upper) rectum to the posterior wall of the urogenital sinus or the vagina, representing the junction of the hindgut with the cloaca (Figs. 3-13G–I and 3-15). This would seem to confirm the origin of the vagina from the urogenital sinus and not from the mülle-

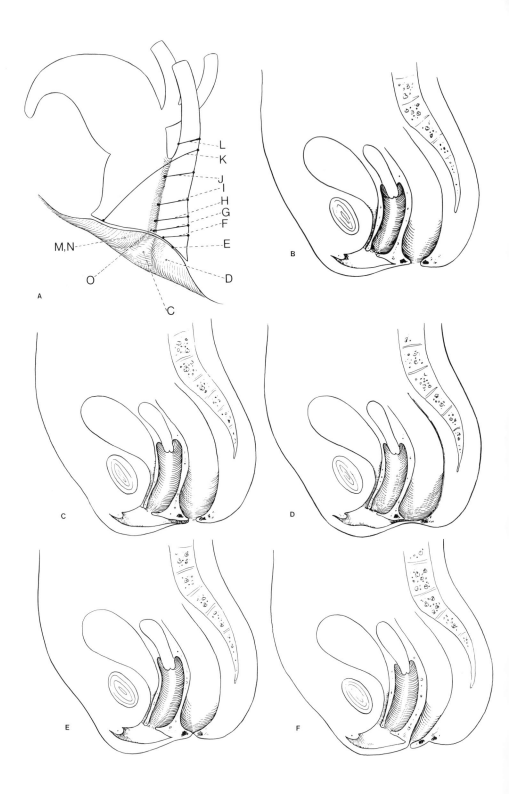

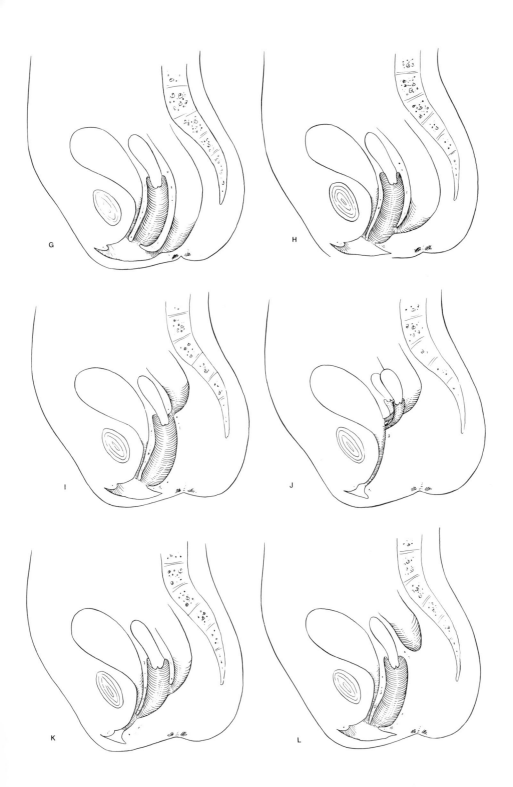

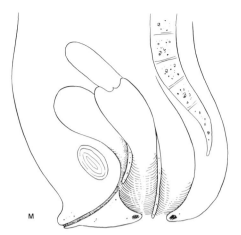

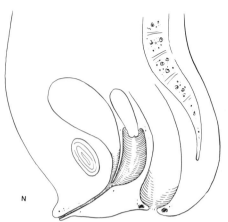

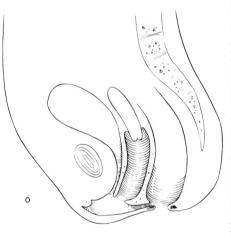

Fig. 3-13. Diagrams of common anomalies of perineum, most of which are associated with excessive resorption of tailgut. *A*. 8-mm embryo. Diagram of cloaca and cloacal membrane in 5-week embryo. The lines C-O indicate the site or extent of the embryonic defect producing the anomalies diagrammed in Figs. 13-*C-O*. The lines F-L indicate the extent of the destruction of the cloaca resulting in the anomalies in Figs. 13-*F-L*. *B*. Normal. *C*. Anofossa navicularis fissure. *D*. Covered anus. *E*. Imperforate anus. *F*. Rectoperineal fistula. *G*. Recto–fossa navicularis fistula. *H*. Rectovaginal fistula, low. *I*. Rectovaginal fistula, high. *J*. Rectovesical fistula. *K*. Recto–urogenital sinus fistula. *L*. Rectal agenesis without fistula. *M*. Posterior displacement of urogenital sinus. *N*. Masculinized female genitalia. *O*. Recto–fossa navicularis fistula with normal anus.

rian ducts as there is never an embryonic connection between the hindgut and the müllerian apparatus.[1] (Persistence of the hindgut-cloacal communication in the male results in rectovesical or rectourethral fistula.)

Rectovesical fistula. Excessive resorption of the cloaca all the way up to the level of the müllerian tubercle may prevent normal fusion of the two müllerian ducts, resulting in two small hemivaginas opening into the base of the bladder on either side of a rectovesical fistula (Figs. 3-13*J*

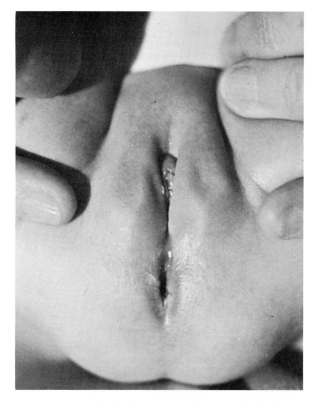

Fig. 3-14. Ano–fossa navicularis fissure extending anteriorly from rectoperineal fistula. This patient has had a cut-back incision from fistula into external anal sphincter.

and 3-16). It should be noted that rectovesical fistula occurs in the female only when the müllerian ducts fail to fuse in the midline above this level.

Recto–urogenital sinus fistula. In some cases with extensive cloacal destruction, the müllerian duct–cloacal junction fails to "descend" to the perineum, probably because the disturbance in development also involves the lower portion of the urogenital sinus as well as the rectal anlage (Fig. 3-13*K*). In this anomaly, there is only one small perineal orifice, near the clitoris, which opens into a long narrow passage receiving first the urethra, then the vagina, and finally the rectum.

Covered anus. Several superficial anomalies of the perineum result from ectodermal and/or mesodermal abnormalities with normal or nearly

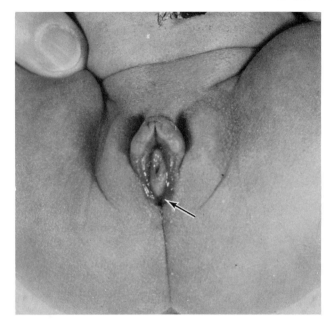

Fig. 3-15. Recto–fossa navicularis fistula (*arrow*) immediately posterior to edematous, protruding hymen of newborn infant.

normal development of the anal membrane and the rectum. A covered anus is one in which a plaque of skin occludes the anal orifice, suggesting a simple fusion of the anal tubercles over a normal anal canal and rectum (Figs. 3-13*D* and 3-17). In this anomaly, which is much more common in the male, there is usually an abnormally prominent midline raphe, alongside of which there are often one or two tiny dimples which may be occluded by a speck of meconium, indicating the lumen of the rectum is just beneath the surface and connected to the exterior by a minute tract.

Ano–fossa navicularis fissure. Failure of midline fusion of the ectoderm over the mesodermal elements of the perineal body results in a shallow mucosa-lined furrow between the anal and urogenital orifices (Figs. 3-13*C*, 3-14, and 3-18). In the female, this ano–fossa navicularis fissure extends anteriorly from either a normal anus or a rectoperineal fistula. This anomaly also is considerably more common in the male, in whom subsequent ectodermal fusion over this furrow may produce a subcutaneous tunnel in the median raphe. The subcutaneous fistula may begin at a normal or an ectopic anus and extend all the way around the scrotum

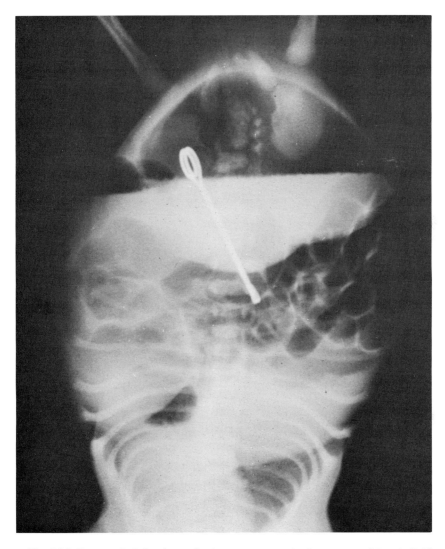

Fig. 3-16. Rectovesical fistula producing pneumocystis, demonstrated by air-fluid level on roentgenogram of newborn in inverted position. There was complete failure of fusion of the two müllerian tubes. Note malformation of sacrum seen through air-filled bladder.

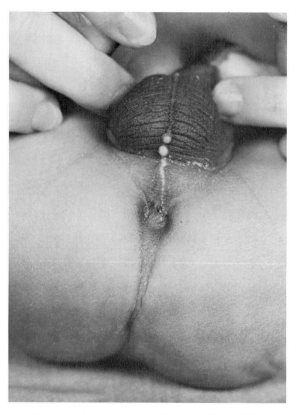

Fig. 3-17. Covered anus with anoscrotal fistula indicated by tiny mucus-filled subcutaneous tract. Plaque of skin covers normal anal canal.

and up to the free edge of the foreskin (Fig. 3-17). A superficial tract is rare in the female.

Recto–fossa navicularis fistula with normal anus. Failure of the uro-rectal fold to descend all the way to the perineum (with normal fusion of the anal tubercles and the labioscrotal folds in the midportion of the cloacal membrane) results in a recto–fossa navicularis fistula with normal anus and rectum (Fig. 3-13O).[5, 26] This is the very rare exception to the rule that there is only one opening in the caudal extremity of the gastrointestinal tract.

Posterior displacement of urogenital sinus. Fusion of the anal tubercle–labioscrotal mesoderm at a site anterior to the location of the urorectal fold combined with fusion of the urethral folds anteriorly is presumed to be the cause of the rare abnormality in which the urogenital sinus has

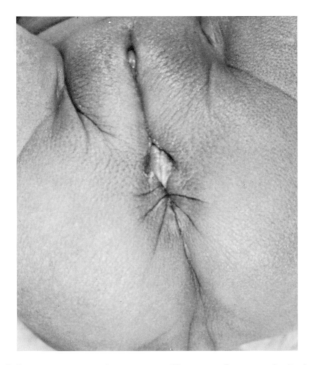

Fig. 3-18. Subcutaneous scarring surrounding ano–fossa navicularis fissure in infant a few weeks old.

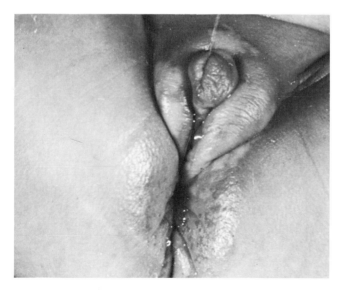

Fig. 3-19. Posterior displacement of urogenital sinus. Patient is voiding a fine stream through stenotic phallic urethra. Depigmentation of skin results from hemangioma already sclerosing spontaneously in this newborn infant.

two external orifices (Fig. 3-13*M*). The "masculine" urethra opens on the tip of the phallus (Fig. 3-19) and the urogenital sinus opens near the anus, within the external anal sphincter (Figs. 3-20 and 3-21). In addition, at the site of the normal female urethra, there is a urethro–urogenital sinus fistula through which most of the fetal urine is voided into the vagina. Constriction of the lower end of the urogenital sinus by the external anal sphincter results in hydrometrocolpos; escape of the urine and genital secretions through the open ends of the fallopian tubes may cause fetal peritonitis.

Masculinization. Embryonic fusion of the urethral folds, similar to that of the preceding anomaly, is part of the pathologic anatomy of the masculinized female with congenital adrenal hyperplasia (Fig. 3-13*N*).

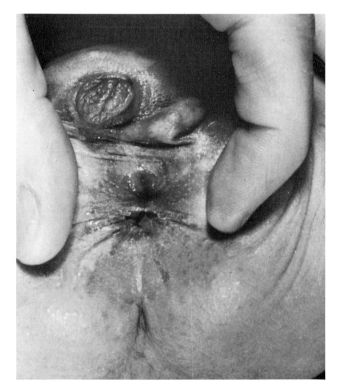

Fig. 3-20. Posterior displacement of urogenital sinus. Eversion of anal canal reveals septum between anus and urogenital sinus, both of which are surrounded by external anal sphincter. Labia are fused in the midline all the way up to phallus. Same patient as Fig. 3-19.

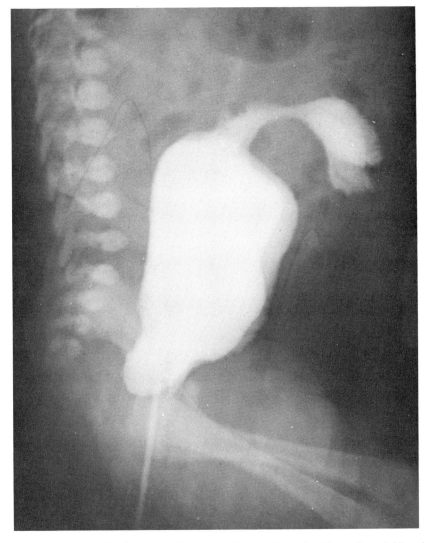

Fig. 3-21. Posterior displacement of urogenital sinus. Note double outline of dilated septate vagina filled with contrast material. Same patient as Fig. 3-19.

In these patients, the vagina usually opens into the masculinized urethra so near the surface of the perineum that a simple cutback vaginoplasty forms a satisfactory external vaginal orifice. In some of these infants, however, the vagina opens into the urethra proximal to the external urethral sphincter, so that a more extensive operative procedure is required to obviate urinary incontinence postoperatively.[15]

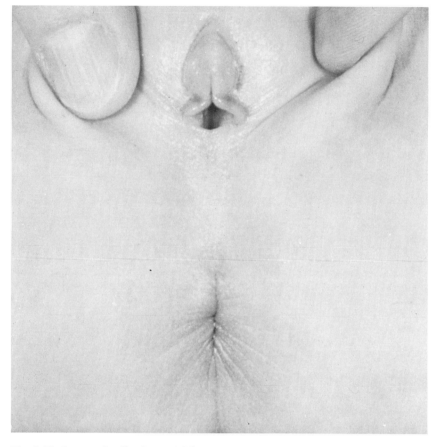

Fig. 3-22. Postnatal adhesions of labia minora covering vaginal orifice in infant a few months old.

This embryonic fusion of the labia is to be differentiated from the postnatal adhesions of the labia minora which follow vulvar irritation or inflammation, usually in a child well past the neonatal period (Fig. 3-22).

Incidence of anorectal and perineal anomalies. The distribution of various types of anorectal and perineal anomalies in the infants at Charity Hospital is questionable, many of the records being incomplete and the description of the pathologic anatomy vague and contradictory. This is a reflection primarily of failure properly to distinguish between rectovaginal and rectofossa navicularis fistula, with the reported incidence too high in the former and too low in the latter. Table 3-1 shows the inci-

TABLE 3-1

ANORECTAL AND PERINEAL ANOMALIES
RELATED TO EMBRYONIC ARREST OR DISTORTION *

Anomaly	Male	Female
Superficial anomalies		
Covered anus	5	
Ano–fossa navicularis fissure		2
Imperforate anus	4	
Intermediate anomalies		
Rectoperineal fistula	5	18
Rectoscrotal fistula	2	
Deep anomalies		
Rectourethral fistula	13	
Recto–fossa navicularis fistula		7
Rectovaginal fistula †		9
Rectovesical fistula	5	1
Rectal agenesis without fistula	2	2
Posterior displacement of urogenital sinus		3
Total	36	42

* These figures do not include patients with exstrophy of the cloaca associated with imperforate anus or males with hypospadias.

† Includes 4 infants with fused labia and 1 with duplication of the external genitalia.

dence of anorectal and perineal anomalies in a comparable series of both private and Charity Hospital patients examined and treated by one of the authors.

Absence of Infraumbilical Abdominal Wall

The abdominal wall is intact, but the lower edge of the umbilicus is only a few millimeters from the external genitalia (Figs. 3-23 and 3-25). Absence of the infraumbilical abdominal wall should be distinguished from gastroschisis, an aperture through the full thickness of the abdominal wall with prenatal evisceration, and from embryonic fissure, an opening into the lumen of the bladder or cloaca. In most cases of embryonic fissure (exstrophy) the defect extends through the infraumbilical abdominal wall from the umbilicus to or into the genitalia.

There were three females and one male with absence of the infraumbilical abdominal wall at Charity Hospital. The male had normal genitalia and anus but died from infection in a lumbar myelomeningocele. Autopsy revealed a small functionless left kidney with absence of the ipsilateral umbilical artery. Two of the females had anorectal agenesis and abnormal fusion of the labioscrotal folds with a normal female

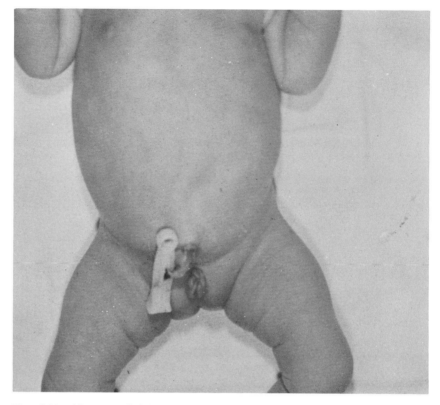

Fig. 3-23. Absence of infraumbilical abdominal wall. Umbilicus arises immediately above external genitalia.

clitoris (Figs. 3-24 and 3-26). Both these infants survived operation for the anorectal anomaly, but one died of renal infection and the other of rupture of an occipital encephalocele. The third female infant had a bifid clitoris but a normal vagina and anus (Fig. 3-11). She survived multiple operations for gastroschisis but had urinary incontinence secondary to associated anomalies of the bladder neck.

Duplication of the External Genitalia

Duplication of the external genitalia is generally thought to be a form of incomplete twinning, but the exact embryologic cause is not known. In many cases the anomaly is compatible with prolonged survival.[29, 34]

The central factor in the doubling process is the cloacal membrane. Division (perforation) of the membrane would produce a fissure through the genital-perineal area and would result in the bifid genitalia seen in

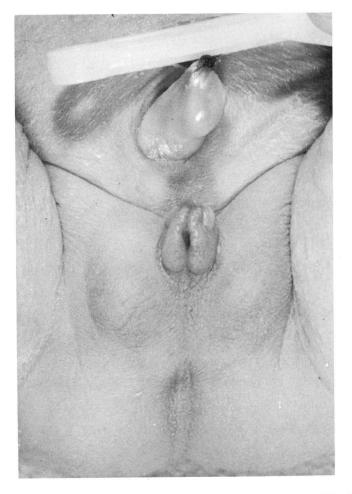

Fig. 3-24. Absence of infraumbilical abdominal wall. Normal umbilical cord arises immediately above abnormally fused labia minora. There was also a recto-vaginal fistula with imperforate anus. Same patient as Fig. 3-23.

exstrophy of the bladder and of the cloaca. True duplication must depend upon two distinct cloacal membranes separated by normal ectoderm and mesoderm. Each then becomes surrounded by normal mesodermal structures (genital tubercle, labioscrotal folds, anal tubercles) and each will be in contact with the endodermal (gut) lumen above. The mesodermal elements between the two membranes might well induce the abnormal sagittal partitioning of the cloaca from below while the urorectal fold partitions in a coronal plane from above. This would account

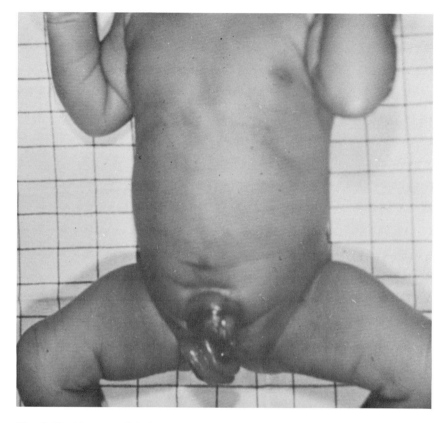

Fig. 3-25. Absence of infraumbilical abdominal wall. Umbilicus arises immediately above external genitalia.

for the doubling of the colon and the bladder usually seen with duplication of the external genitalia.

Evidence that this duplication is a caudal process is found in the derivatives of the urogenital ridge (wolffian and müllerian ducts) which are normally paired and not quadruple. The kidneys are usually normal, with one ureter draining into each bladder, and there are generally two ovaries and two fallopian tubes, each attached to a unicornuate uterus opening into a vagina in each set of genitalia. If two embryos were superimposed upon one another, as has been suggested, might not each bladder be expected to have two ureters?

The variations in the pathologic anatomy suggest that either anterior or posterior bifurcation of the cloacal membrane can occur. This would account for a single clitoris with double labia and a double anus, or a

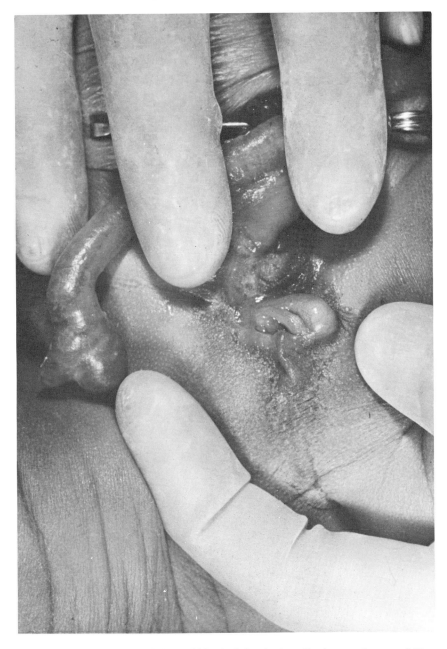

Fig. 3-26. Absence of infraumbilical abdominal wall. A prominent midline raphe indicates fusion of labia immediately beneath umbilicus containing supernumerary loop of bowel. Same patient as Fig. 3-25.

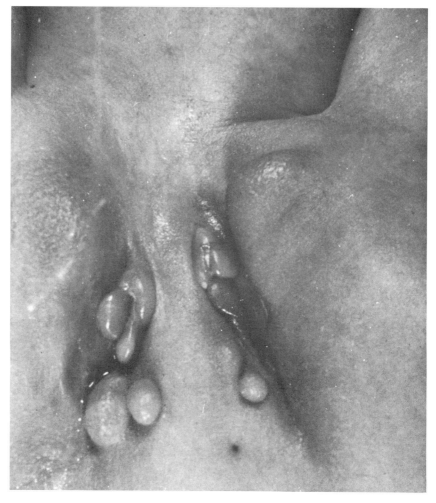

Fig. 3-27. Duplication of external genitalia. CH64-81026. Note two normal labia majora laterally and two medial labia majora represented by polypoid masses. Each clitoris has two labia minora surrounding a normal vagina. The two dimples represent two imperforate ani.

double clitoris and double labia with a single anus. It would also explain the variability in doubling of the lower vertebral column and the spinal cord.

Duplication of the genitalia (Fig. 3-27) should be distinguished from (1) the bifid phallus and the unfused labioscrotal folds occurring with embryonic fissure (exstrophy) (Figs. 3-7 through 3-10) and (2) the doubling of the genitalia seen in conjoined twins (Figs. 3-30 and 3-32). In this latter condition, the external genitalia can be expected to be aligned properly with the symphysis pubis, even though the symphysis marks the midlateral line of junction of the two trunks and not the anterior midline of either twin.

One case of duplication of the external genitalia and two of female conjoined twins occurred in the Charity Hospital admissions.

Duplication of the external genitalia. CH64-81026. The patient was referred because of an imperforate anus and a large myelomeningocele. Examination revealed imperfect duplication of the genitalia, the medial labium majus on each side being distorted into polypoid masses

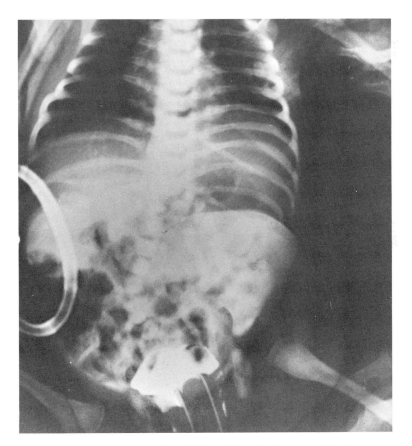

Fig. 3-28. Duplication of genitalia. CH64-81026. Bladders are filled by catheters in two urethras. Note bifid lumbosacral vertebral column.

(Fig. 3-27). There were two imperforate ani and a high rectovaginal fistula to the right vagina. The lower vertebral column was bifid, beginning at L1 (Fig. 3-28). At the time of colostomy, exploration of the abdomen revealed two urinary bladders and two widely separated unicornuate uteri with normal tubes and ovaries. The single colon had a double blood supply with a mesentery attached to each lateral wall of the pelvis. The child survived the immediate postoperative period but was lost to follow-up after discharge from the hospital.

Duplication of the perineum in conjoined twins. CH55-181542. This ischiopagus conjoined twin had one bony pelvic ring formed from the conjoined pelvic girdles of the two infants (Fig. 3-29). The two complete sets of external and internal genitalia were in proper relation to

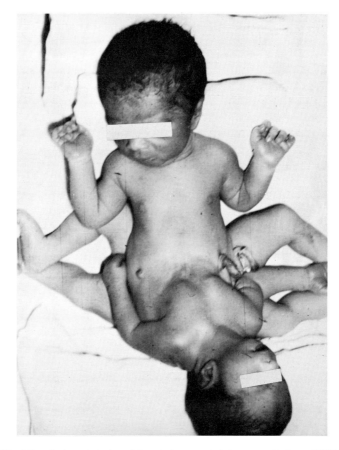

Fig. 3-29. Dicephalus tetrabrachius tetrapus ischiopagus twins. CH55-181542.
(From Spencer, R. *Surgery* 39:827, 1956.)

the two symphyses pubis (Fig. 3-30), disregarding the fact that each infant contributed one pubic ramus to each symphysis. On the side of the perineum near the larger twin was a midline fissure with no internal connection (an abortive attempt at anus formation); on the side near the smaller infant was a small open anus without a sphincter. At operation, two urinary bladders and two uteri were shared by both infants. One ureter of each child drained into each bladder, and one tube of each uterus extended into the pelvis of each child. The single colon opened into the incontinent anal orifice.

The nonviable parasitic twin was separated from the larger, more normal infant. The entire anterior abdominal wall with two umbilici and the entire conjoined perineum were used to close the abdomen of the surviving twin. This infant was left with a complete gastrointestinal tract with one perforate and one imperforate anus; two kidneys, each draining into a separate bladder; two uteri with four tubes

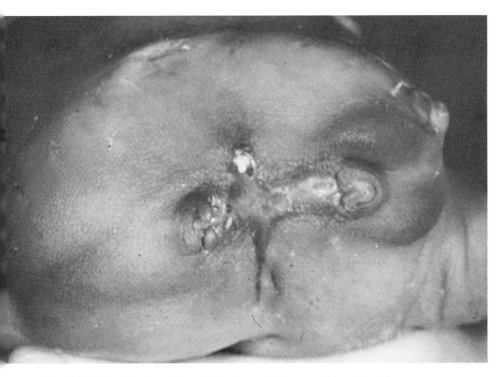

Fig. 3-30. Duplication of genitalia in surviving member of ischiopagus conjoined twins. CH55-181542. The two normal sets of genitalia were aligned at right angles to the two pubic symphyses. Single anus is indicated by speck of light-colored feces.

and ovaries; and three vaginas, the genitalia on the left side having a septate vagina.

Intravenous pyelography at age 11 years revealed normal urinary tracts.

Duplication of the perineum with conjoined twins. CH68-182051. These dicephalus tripus tribrachius twins were stillborn (Fig. 3-31). There was an almost symmetrical lateral duplication of the external genitalia (Fig. 3-32) but anterior-posterior duplication of the internal genitalia,

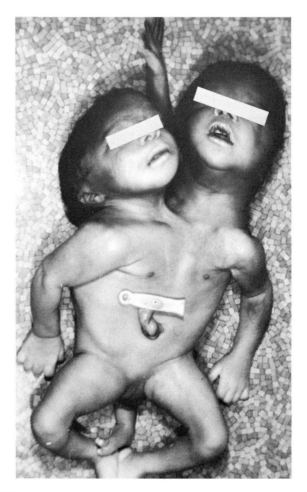

Fig. 3-31. Dicephalus tripus tribrachius thoraco-omphalopagus twins. CH68-182051.

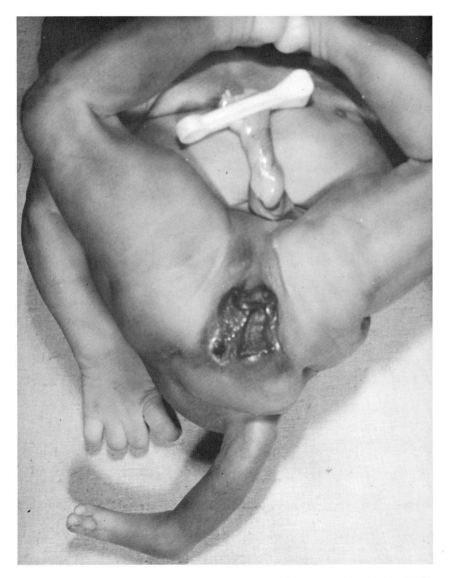

Fig. 3-32. Duplication of genitalia in thoraco-omphalopagus twins. CH68-182051. A third leg emerges from posterior aspect of trunk.

the posterior viscera being small and distorted and opening to the left external genitalia.

MALFORMATIONS OF THE INTERNAL GENITALIA

Isolated anomalies of the internal genitalia are diagnosed in infancy and childhood only incidentally at laparotomy for other disease. Since these viscera have no primary function before puberty, no physiologic derangement accompanies anatomic abnormality, nor does obstruction usually become manifest since there is little or no secretion or effusion into the prepubertal female genital tract. However, abnormalities of the internal genitalia frequently accompany anomalies of other pelvic viscera, hence discovery of an anomaly in any one of these organs indicates investigation of the status of the others.

Gonads

The development of the ovary is completely independent of that of the müllerian ducts, and while the exact origin of the germ cells may be in doubt, it is apparent that the ovarian stroma can develop even in the absence of the germ cells. Thus a defect in one of these elements—germ cells, ovaries, or müllerian ducts—does not necessarily affect the development of the others.

Gonadal Dysgenesis (Bonnevie-Ullrich or Turner's Syndrome)

There are no germ cells in the fibrous ovary which consists of a long thin streak of tissue attached to the broad ligament parallel to the fallopian tube. Since the external genitalia in these patients are usually those of a normal female, the diagnosis is not made in infancy unless there are associated somatic abnormalities. (The occasional patient with gonadal dysgenesis who has clitoral hypertrophy, presumably due to an abundance of Leydig cells in the ovarian streak, must be investigated as an intersex problem.)

With increasing awareness of all the various clinical manifestations, gonadal dysgenesis is being recognized more frequently in the newborn period. The most consistent sign at this age is edema of the dorsum of the hands and feet, usually associated with shortness of the neck.[30] The birth weight is generally low, even after full-term gestation. There is usually some degree of webbing of the neck, and often low-set ears, micrognathia, and an abnormal whorled pattern of the hair at the base of the skull. Other somatic manifestations likely to be noted in infancy include high arched palate, cubitus valgus, syndactyly, cardiovascular

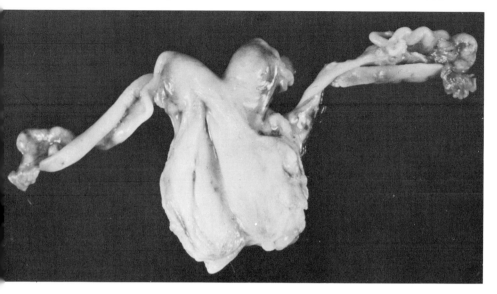

Fig. 3-33. Very elongated ovaries and bicornuate ovaries in a newborn. These ovaries contained normal ova. (Courtesy of Dr. Ambrose Hertzog, New Orleans.)

defects (most commonly coarctation of the aorta [13]), and a high incidence of urinary tract anomalies.[18]

Even though the infant appears to be a normal female, buccal smear may show a male nuclear chromatin pattern, and karyotyping reveals an abnormality in the sex chromosomes (X monosomy). Laparotomy is not indicated for diagnosis, but examination of the internal genitalia would reveal a normal uterus and fallopian tubes, but streak ovaries without germ cells or follicular elements. Small cysts of the rete ovarii should not be mistakenly identified as follicular cysts; the rete tubules and remnants of the mesonephric duct and tubules are normally present in these patients.[9] Also, the fetal shape of the gonad alone is not diagnostic of abnormality (Fig. 3-33), for the ovary is often considerably elongated rather than rounded in early infancy, and a streak ovary in the newborn period may contain normal ova (Fig. 3-34).

The Charity Hospital cases of gonadal dysgenesis are discussed in Chapter Five.

Ovarian Agenesis

Neither absence nor abnormality of the ovary usually accompanies absence of the fallopian tube, but it has been suggested [25] that absence of one ovary and tube may be the result of torsion and infarction during

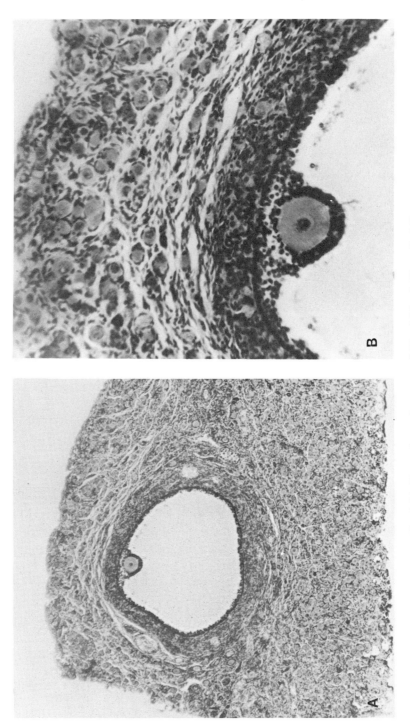

Fig. 3-34. Normal ova in ovary of Fig. 3-33. *A.* 70×, *B.* 240×.

intrauterine life. In such a case, the fundus of the uterus should have a normal configuration and not the conical shape of the unicornuate uterus which develops solely from one müllerian duct.

There is no documented case of absence of one or both ovaries diagnosed in infancy or childhood in the Charity Hospital material.

Cysts and Tumors

Cysts, usually only a few millimeters in diameter, occur in the ovary at any age, even during fetal life. They are assumed to indicate the presence of normal germ cells with developing follicles, but they may be found in the gonads of patients with gonadal dysgenesis.

Cysts or tumors large enough to produce symptoms—or even to be detected on physical examination—are rare in early infancy but have been reported in the newborn.[41] Most are simple follicular or theca lutein cysts; very few are neoplastic cysts or solid tumors.[20,22] Functioning tumors are still more rare.

The ovaries are normally high in the pelvis in early infancy, and the small size and the narrow configuration of the infant pelvis encourages an enlarging ovary to rise into the abdominal cavity above. Consequently, ovarian cysts and tumors are more likely to be found in the lower abdomen than in the pelvis of an infant.[2] They may be found on routine abdominal palpation or when abdominal enlargement develops. Infrequently, torsion of the ovary enlarged by a cyst causes acute abdominal symptoms necessitating emergency laparotomy.

Ovarian teratoma, usually cystic, is not uncommon in childhood, but is rarely diagnosed in infancy. The youngest child with a teratoma was 21 months old when she was admitted to Charity Hospital with torsion and infarction of the ovary containing the teratoma.

Grossly cystic ovaries have been reported, usually associated with maternal diabetes or toxemia.[14] Since apparently these ovaries can gradually resume a normal size and configuration if the infant survives, oophorectomy is not indicated for cystic ovaries in the newborn period.[21]

Ovarian cyst in infancy. Touro Infirmary No. 66-005822. This 2-month-old white infant developed a temperature of 102° F, had several loose stools, and required medication for "colic." There was no anorexia or vomiting. The next day the symptoms persisted and a pediatrician found a cystic mass in the abdomen.

On examination the infant seemed to be in mild shock. There was a spherical mass in the right lower quadrant, the mobility of which could not be determined because of marked tenderness of the mass. The remainder of the abdomen was soft and not tender, but the peristalsis was hyperactive because of the gastroenteritis. The mass could not be felt per rectum.

At operation on the day of admission, a 5.5-cm cyst was found in the right ovary. The ovary and the tube had twisted 360° and were infarcted. One hemostat was clamped across the area of torsion, the tube and ovary excised, and the pedicle ligated. The other tube and ovary and the uterus were normal. Recovery was uneventful and the infant was discharged from the hospital 72 hours after operation.

Histologic examination revealed this to be a simple cyst, the lining of which had been destroyed. The tube and ovary showed early infarction, but there was no evidence of neoplasm or embryonic tissue.

Gonadal Ectopia

Ectopia is less common in the female than in the male. The gonads arise near the mesonephric ridge, superior to the origin of the metanephros (the definitive human kidney), and descend into the lower portion of the abdominal cavity during early fetal life. Arrest of descent at this early stage will leave the gonad (either testis or ovary) in the embryonic position high in the abdomen.[19, 24]

A few weeks before birth the testes leave the abdomen and go into the scrotum. Just as the testis may be arrested at any point on its journey, so can the ovary travel too far. At the time the processus vaginalis develops, the testis and the ovary occupy the same intraabdominal position and have the same opportunity to prolapse into the inguinal canal. The testis normally does so before birth, and if an inguinal hernia develops in the first few months of extrauterine life, the ovary will normally be found in the patent processus vaginalis (Fig. 3-35). With increasing age, the pelvis becomes broader and deeper, the normal position of the ovary moves farther from the internal ring, and the presence of the ovary in the hernia sac becomes less frequent.

The ovary is also said to occur outside the external ring without a hernia sac, but this must be a very rare finding.[17]

The mere presence of an ovary in a hernia sac in a female infant with normal external genitalia is no cause for alarm and does not indicate a need for chromosome karyotyping or hormonal assay. However, should any abnormality be noted during hernia repair, the incision can be enlarged, the internal genitalia examined, and the gonads biopsied.[12] Other investigation can then be completed postoperatively.

Splenogonadal Fusion

This is a rare anomaly resulting from the embryonic adhesion of the spleen to the left gonad. This undoubtedly occurs during the sixth to

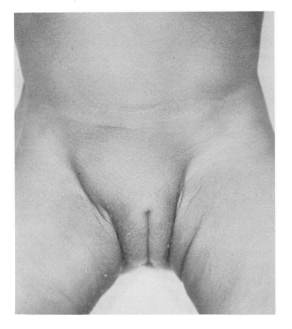

Fig. 3-35. Inguinal hernia containing incarcerated (but not strangulated) ovary in 7-week-old baby.

the eighth week of embryogenesis, when the spleen is forming in the dorsal mesogastrium immediately adjacent to the gonadal ridge. Later, when the gonad descends, a cord of fibrous and/or splenic tissue forms between the two viscera, usually traversing the free peritoneal cavity and often interfering with the descent of the gonad and closure of the processus vaginalis. Less commonly, a separate nodule of splenic tissue accompanies the gonad to its definitive position in the pelvis or the scrotum (discontinuous fusion).

There are only 4 female patients in the 53 cases of splenogonadal fusion reported in the literature.[33, 40] Three newborn female infants all had continuous fusion which prevented complete ovarian descent; two had multiple congenital anomalies. The fourth patient, an adult female with a septate uterus, had a 1.5-cm cluster of splenic nodules on the left ovary.

Supernumerary Ovaries

The finding of extra ovarian tissue, as an organ or a nodule, is quite rare, only 4 documented cases having been reported.[42] Accessory ovarian tissue near the main ovary is only slightly more common (19 cases reported).[32, 42] There was no case of splenogonadal fusion or of supernumerary or accessory ovary among Charity Hospital patients.

Genital Canal

The genital canal in the female has its origin in the paired müllerian (paramesonephric) ducts which arise on the posterior abdominal wall lateral to the mesonephric ducts. The midportion of the ducts meet in the midline and fuse to form a single structure which acquires an external opening in the urogenital sinus below. Anomalies of the genital canal include (1) agenesis of all or part of one or both müllerian ducts, (2) imperfect fusion of the two ducts, and (3) incomplete canalization.

The development of the müllerian ducts is more closely related to that of the mesonephric ducts than to that of the ovaries. Consequently anomalies of the genital canal are associated with anomalies of the kidney and ureter more frequently than with abnormalities of the ovaries. Also, the genital canal may be quite normal in gonadal dysgenesis, but the upper urinary tract is likely to be abnormal.[18]

Absence of the Müllerian Apparatus

Agenesis is usually found only in fetuses without upper urinary tracts. Absence of one duct results in a unicornuate uterus, and absence of a portion of a duct results in a short fallopian tube with little or no connection to the normal component on the other side (Fig. 3-36). In both these latter cases, there is a high incidence of absence or abnormality of the ipsilateral kidney and ureter,[45] but the ovaries can be expected to be normal.[45] Absence of (all or) most of both ducts would result in absence of the uterus with an "empty" broad ligament between the two ovaries.[3]

Müllerian duct agenesis. CH57-276118. The only Charity Hospital case reported to have absence of the genital canal is open to question because various entries in the record are conflicting.

A 5-year-old girl admitted for incontinence was found to have external genitalia normal except for some enlargement of the labia. The urethra was patent and the 3-cm vagina was "open." In addition, there was a "vesicovaginal fistula" with "absence of the septum between the vagina and the bladder."

At operation the left kidney was found to be absent (but the ureter present) and both ovaries were identified. At a subsequent operation only the left ovary was found. The uterus and (upper) vagina were

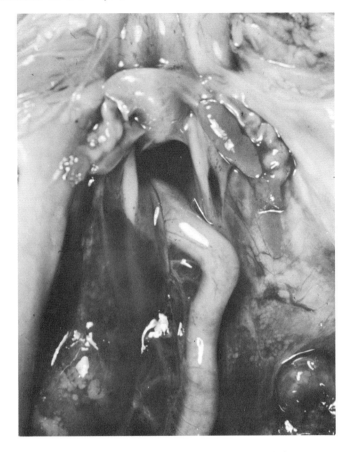

Fig. 3-36. Unicornuate uterus resulting from absence of right cornu. Tortuous
fallopian tubes and elongated ovaries are normal in newborn.

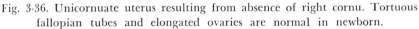

noted to be absent. The bladder was excised and an ileal loop constructed for urinary diversion.

It is noteworthy that no mention was made of fallopian tubes or round
or broad ligaments. The small unfused müllerian ducts in a prepubertal
child may well be overlooked, particularly when attention was focused
on the urinary tract rather than the genital canal. The short vagina
opening on the perineum is assumed to be of urogenital sinus origin.

Unilateral absence of the müllerian duct. CH60-365893. A poorly described case of unilateral absence of the müllerian duct and ovary

occurred in a stillborn who also had absence of both kidneys and bladder, imperforate anus, atresia of the larynx, and left anophthalmia. Surprisingly, the external genitalia were described as normal!

Partial absence of one müllerian duct. Touro Infirmary No. 69-078718. A 3-lb infant who had imperforate anus with a recto–fossa navicularis fistula succumbed of pneumonitis 10 days after correction of duodenal atresia. Autopsy revealed two normal tubes and ovaries with a unicornuate uterus (Fig. 3-36), normal kidneys, and absence of the gallbladder and the interatrial septum.

The upper portion of the genital canal (the müllerian ducts) may be normal but the lower segment missing, as though the müllerian contribution failed to connect properly with the urogenital sinus. This may result in absence of all or part of the vagina and is one of the few anomalies of the internal genitalia which is in itself likely to produce enough symptoms to be diagnosed in infancy (absence of the vagina with hydrometra). In a few instances, the rudimentary short vagina opening on the perineum represents the contribution of the urogenital sinus to the female genital tract.

Absence of the vagina. CH53-104084. Autopsy on a 5-day-old anuric baby revealed absence of the vagina, cystic dilation of the uterus and cervix, absence of the left kidney and ureter, polycystic right kidney, and hypoplasia of the urinary bladder. There was no mention of the external genitalia.

Imperfect Fusion of Müllerian Ducts

The most common anomalies of the internal genitalia, imperfect fusion produces defects ranging from septate and bicornuate uterus through uterus didelphys with septate vagina. The bipartite structures occupy a normal position in the pelvis and the ease of diagnosis depends on the extent of the external separation, the most severe being recognized by simple inspection. Incomplete fusion is diagnosed in infancy and childhood only incidentally at autopsy or during operation for other conditions.

In this series, there were only three infants (CH58-312148, CH50-425015, and CH49-379914, all autopsy cases) who were recognized to have "bifid" or bicornuate uterus without abnormalities of the perineum and/or external genitalia. It is significant that all three had abnormalities of the upper urinary tracts (cystic, polycystic, or horseshoe kidney) as well as abnormalities in other parts of the body (diaphragmatic hernia, hydrocephaly, polydactyly, biliary atresia), but the ovaries were normal. The apparent scarcity of these conditions probably indicates that instances of isolated septate vagina and bicornuate uterus escaped detection in infants without other genitourinary abnormalities.

Bicornuate uterus with abnormal external genitalia. CH65-90731. A full-term white female infant with imperforate anus had wide separation of the labia majora. The urethral and vaginal orifices were surrounded by tiny labia minora which were fused together posteriorly (Fig. 3-24). The normal umbilical cord arose only a few millimeters above the external genitalia (absence of the infraumbilical abdominal wall, Fig. 3-23) and there was a palpable diastasis pubis. At operation she was found to have a bicornuate uterus with a high rectovaginal fistula into the single vagina. The ovaries were normal. Also noted were bilateral hydronephrosis and hydroureter and a Meckel's diverticulum. The infant died of pyelonephritis 10 days after suprapubic cystostomy and abdominoperineal repair of the imperforate anus.

If the müllerian ducts fail to meet at all in the midline, the two small unicornuate uteri and hemivaginas will be situated quite laterally and superiorly in the pelvis, near the internal inguinal ring, and may be identified only by their proximity to the ovary and continuity with the fallopian tube. The unicornuate uterus constitutes a conical thickening in the midportion of the "tube" with a thinner distal portion representing the hemivagina. The vaginal extremity of the duct rarely (if ever) reaches the perineum, and there are often defects of the cloacal derivatives into which they empty. Complete failure of fusion of the müllerian ducts is rarely seen as an isolated anomaly but frequently accompanies anomalies of other pelvic viscera.

Bilateral unicornuate uterus with abnormal external genitalia. CH60-345686. A newborn female infant with imperforate anus had fused labia, minimal enlargement of the clitoris, and a small urethral meatus. When she was 24 hours old the abdomen was tremendously distended but thin-walled because of "absence" of the abdominal musculature. X-rays showed pneumo- and megacystis (Fig. 3-16). At operation the müllerian ducts were found to be completely unfused, with two small hemivaginas opening into the base of the bladder on either side of a rectovesical fistula. The ovaries were normal, but the kidneys were cystic and hydronephrotic, and the ureters and bladder tremendously dilated. Malrotation and Hirschsprung's disease were two incidental findings. Transverse colostomy and suprapubic cystostomy were done, and the infant died of uremia at the age of 16 days. At autopsy evidence of prenatal peritonitis (cornified squamous epithelial cells on the serosal surfaces of the viscera) was thought to have resulted from escape of urine and vaginal fluid through the open ends of the fallopian tubes.

The findings in this case illustrate the fact that it is only when the two fallopian tubes fail to meet in the midline that rectovesical fistula occurs in the female with imperforate anus (see under Embryonic Arrest or Distortion).

Complete failure of fusion of the müllerian ducts must be differentiated from incomplete fusion with the two vaginal canals enclosed in a common fascial sheath (septate vagina). With complete failure of fusion, the orifices of the two müllerian ducts will rarely reach the perineum, so the external genitalia will be grossly abnormal. In a septate vagina with a common fascial sheath, the external genitalia will appear normal to casual inspection, and it is only when the labia are separated that the vaginal septum will be seen.

Septate vagina with normal external genitalia. CH60-360647. A full-term white female infant with imperforate anus had normal external genitalia. X-rays showed lumbar hemivertebrae. At operation a bicornuate uterus was found atop a septate vagina, with a high rectovaginal fistula to the right vagina. The left kidney was polycystic and the ureter atretic; the right was normal. During abdominoperineal repair of the imperforate anus, the lower edge of the complete longitudinal vaginal septum could be seen from the perineum. The infant survived operation but was lost to follow-up after discharge from the hospital.

Two other infants with imperforate anus and normal external genitalia had uterus didelphys with septate vagina. One (CH43-95161) had successful repair of the imperforate anus but died after operation for atresia of the esophagus. The other (CH49-378490), who also had harelip and cleft palate, survived operation for an omphalocele, then died after colostomy for the imperforate anus. She was found at autopsy also to have congenital heart disease (tetralogy of Fallot).

Septate vagina with abnormal genitalia. CH64-75585. A Negro female infant with imperforate anus had wide separation of the labia majora and no visible clitoris or vagina (Fig. 3-26). There was only one perineal orifice, apparently urethra, surrounded by the labia minora, which were fused together posteriorly. In addition, there were an occipital encephalocele and a small omphalocele from which protruded the blind end of a small segment of bowel. The umbilicus was only a few millimeters above the abnormal genitalia (absence of the infraumbilical abdominal wall; Fig. 3-25), and beneath the thin skin in this area, a pubic diastasis was palpable.

At operation, a uterus didelphys was found above a septate vagina. The rectum did open through a minute orifice on the perineum, just posterior to the vaginal septum (recto–fossa navicularis fistula). The orifice of the septate vagina was found between the labia minora and behind the urethra. The intestine in the umbilicus had no internal connection and was assumed to be of omphalomesenteric duct origin. Abdominoperineal operation was successfully completed, but the infant died when the encephalocele ruptured on the sixth postoperative day.

Incomplete Canalization of Genital Canal (Including Hymen)

This is the only isolated congenital abnormality of the reproductive tract which is likely to produce enough symptoms to be diagnosed in infancy or early childhood. The ensuing obstruction prevents escape of the endocervical gland secretions which are produced in the neonatal period as a result of stimulation by maternal estrogen.

Incomplete canalization results in three types of obstruction: (1) imperforate hymen, (2) transverse septum of the vagina, and (3) atresia or absence of (all or part of) the vagina (Fig. 3-37). The time of onset and the severity of the symptoms vary with the amount of secretion accumulated in the upper portion of the genital tract and with the degree of obstruction produced in the adjacent viscera by the enlarging vagina and/or uterus.[36]

The proximity of the vagina to the iliac vessels, the rectum, the urethra, and the ureters explains the variety of presenting symptoms in these infants: circulatory, intestinal, or urinary obstruction, usually the latter. The most striking physical finding is the firm, smooth mass arising from the pelvis and occasionally reaching as high as the costal margin. This mass is the vagina itself, tremendously enlarged, containing as much as a liter of cloudy, mucoid fluid. It may seem to be lobulated because of a distended bladder anteriorly, hydronephrotic kidneys laterally, and a moderately enlarged uterus superiorly.

The three lesions which produce hydrometrocolpos can be differentiated by examination of the perineum. A bulging mass protruding

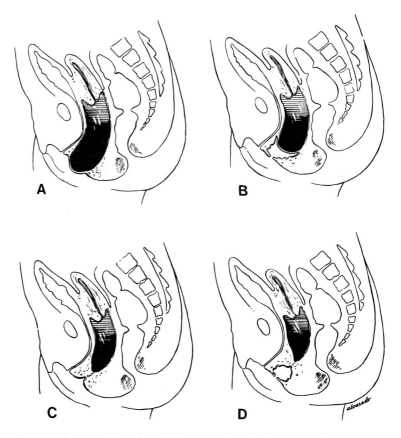

Fig. 3-37. Diagram of various lesions causing hydrometrocolpos. *A*. Imperforate hymen. *B*. Transverse septum. *C* and *D*. Low and high astresia of vagina. (From Spencer, R., and Levy, D. M. *Ann Surg 155*:558, 1962.)

through the labia is usually an imperforate hymen under pressure from the accumulated secretions in the vagina (Fig. 3-38), but careful examination may reveal the rim of a normal hymen displaced peripherally by a transverse septum bulging down from above. In these instances (imperforate hymen and transverse septum), the vulva may be engorged and edematous as a result of local venous and lymphatic engorgement.

With atresia of the vagina ("absence of the lower vagina"), separation of the labia majora will reveal that the structures derived from the urogenital sinus (urethra, vaginal orifice, vestibule) are retracted out of sight up into the pelvis, the result of the upward pull of the enlarging vagina

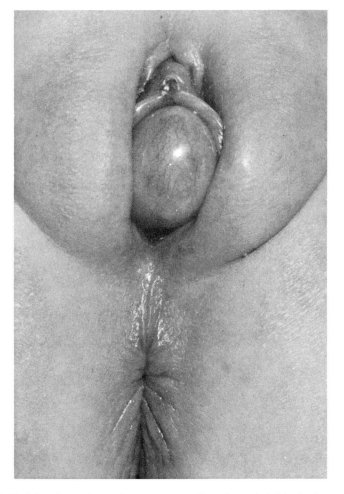

Fig. 3-38. Bulging imperforate hymen protruding through labia in 2-month-old baby with hydrometrocolpos. (Photographed by Dr. Bert Myers.)

escaping from the small pelvis into the spacious abdominal cavity above (Fig. 3-39). Rarely, a high transverse septum may do the same, but most high septa are incomplete and therefore will not cause obstruction at this age.

Atresia of the vagina with hydrometrocolpos. CH58-284210. A Negro female infant who had had abdominal distention since birth was admitted at 3 months of age because of urinary tract infection and

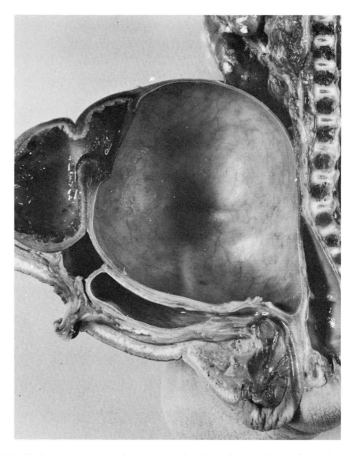

Fig. 3-39. Hydrometrocolpos due to atresia of vagina, with moderately enlarged
uterus above very distended vagina. Ch62-259481.

obstruction. The infant was acutely ill and obviously uncomfortable,
with a firm, smooth mass occupying the entire lower abdomen and
extending almost to the costal margin. The labia were normal, but
the area of the urethral and vaginal orifices was retracted upward out
of sight. By using an otoscope as a speculum, the urethral meatus was
found to be normal. There was no hymen, but the location of the
atretic vagina was indicated by a deep dimple.

X-rays showed bilateral hydronephrosis and hydroureter with anterior and superior displacement of the bladder (Fig. 3-40). A long
narrow urachal tract prolapsed through an umbilical hernia.

Using an abdominoperineal approach, the vagina was emptied of

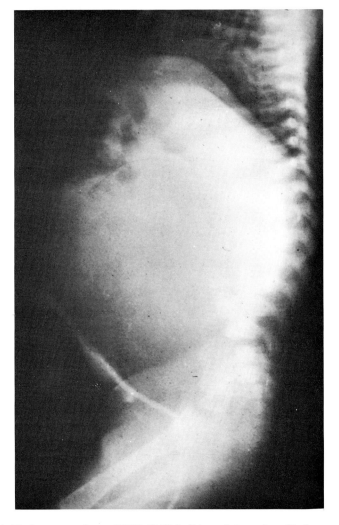

Fig. 3-40 Hydrometrocolpos. CH58-284210. Distended vagina displaces contrast-filled bladder anteriorly and small intestine superiorly.

800 ml of foul mucoid fluid and then opened onto the perineum. Postoperatively, the orifice was maintained by periodic dilation until healing was complete.

Atresia of the vagina with hydrometrocolpos. CH59-314602. A 5-month-old Negro girl who was admitted in congestive failure due to congenital heart disease, had been noted to draw up her legs and strain as if to expel flatus. She cried when she voided, and the urine had a foul odor.

The genitalia were described as normal, but it required at least three attempts before the urethra could be located for catheterization. X-rays showed obstructive uropathy. The urologist noted at cystoscopy that "the bladder is pushed forward for some reason" and on digital rectal examination found a cystic mass anterior to the rectum. A mass was then felt in the lower abdomen. A gynecology consultant was unable to locate the vaginal aperture.

At operation a 5-cm cystic mass was found between the uterus and the rectum, extending to the pelvic peritoneum and intimately adherent to the uterus and bladder. After 20 ml of foul cloudy fluid was aspirated, the mass was opened and the smooth fibrous wall biopsied. The operative diagnosis was "cystic degeneration of an inoperable malignancy."

The cyst fluid contained red and white blood cells, cornified epithelial cells, and Döderlein's bacilli, but no malignant cells. The pathologist reported "stratified squamous and glandular epithelium overlying dense fibromuscular tissue containing a chronic inflammatory infiltrate." No malignancy was seen.

Postoperatively the infant remained febrile. The abdominal mass continued to enlarge until it appeared to be about to drain spontaneously through the perineum, when a stab wound in the area normally occupied by the vaginal orifice evacuated 3–4 oz of purulent fluid. In spite of repeated dilations of the opening and aspiration of the fluid, the urinary tract obstruction continued and hysterectomy was considered. When the dilator was finally successfully passed into the "cyst," fluid ceased to accumulate in the cavity and the urinary tract slowly returned to normal.

Another infant (CH62-259481) with vaginal atresia (Fig. 3-39) died at the age of 24 hours from respiratory distress syndrome in spite of transabdominal aspiration of most of the vaginal fluid.

Lesser degrees of hydrometrocolpos resulted from imperforate hymen in two infants. One was recognized at birth and the other at 2 months of age (Fig. 3-38), when a bulging mass protruded from the labia. Both were relieved of obstruction by a simple linear incision in the hymen without anesthesia.

Cystic Vestiges

During the second month, the embryo possesses the anatomic potential to develop into either sex, the rudiments of the genital tract for both sexes being present in all embryos. After the second month, the genital tract appropriate for the chromosomal sex of the embryo continues to grow and differentiate, while the ductal system for the opposite sex ceases to develop and begins to disintegrate.

The female müllerian (paramesonephric) ducts are specifically designed to become a genital tract. The male, having no structures destined for this purpose, appropriates the discarded mesonephric (wolffian) duct and tubules which become useless to the urinary tract as soon as the metanephros develops.

Both sexes retain vestiges of the discarded cranial portion of the mesonephric system; in addition the male also has remnants of the primitive female genital tract.

In the female, mesonephric duct remnants occur along a line extending from the fimbriated end of the fallopian tube, through the broad ligament parallel to the fallopian tube, lateral to or through the muscular wall of the uterus and cervix, and anterolaterally in the vagina.[10] Stalked vesicles associated with the fimbriated end of the fallopian tube or in the adjacent broad ligament are the hydatids of Morgagni, the blind cranial end of the mesonephric duct. Between the fallopian tube and the ovary is the epoophoron (parovarium, organ of Rosenmüller), a single longitudinal duct in the mesosalpinx communicating with several smaller tubules in the mesovarium; these structures represent the main mesonephric duct and the vertical mesonephric tubules, respectively. More caudal mesonephric tubules in the broad ligament between the ovary and the uterus are known as the paroophoron, and further distally, alongside the uterus and vagina, the mesonephric duct becomes Gartner's duct.[43]

Imperfect canalization of the müllerian (paramesonephric) apparatus may result in small remnants in these same locations, and cystic vestiges in the mesovarium can also arise from the rete ovarii in the hilum of the ovary.

Intraabdominal cystic vestiges are rarely found in infancy. Vaginal cysts do occur, although infrequently. Differential diagnosis, usually not important clinically, depends upon location and histology.[10] Mesonephric duct cysts always occur along the anterolateral sides of the vagina.[17] Müllerian (paramesonephric) duct cysts are also found in this location but are more common near the cervix; they may show histologic structure corresponding to that of the tubes, endometrium, cervix, or vagina, and may contain mucus but do not possess a basement membrane. The mesonephric duct cysts do not show secretory activity but have a basement membrane.[16]

Urethral cysts—obstructed, dilated periurethral glands—may develop in the urethrovaginal septum and bulge the anterior wall of the vagina or protrude into the vaginal vestibule (Fig. 3-41).

Anomalous localized overgrowth of the anterior vaginal wall may produce a mass protruding between the labia (Fig. 3-42*A*). Histologic study reveals fibroconnective tissue stroma, an epithelial covering, and a few mucous crypts of the type found in the periurethral gland (Fig. 3-42*B*).

The importance of this malformation is that it resembles, clinically, the polypoid growth of a malignant neoplasm, sarcoma botryoides.

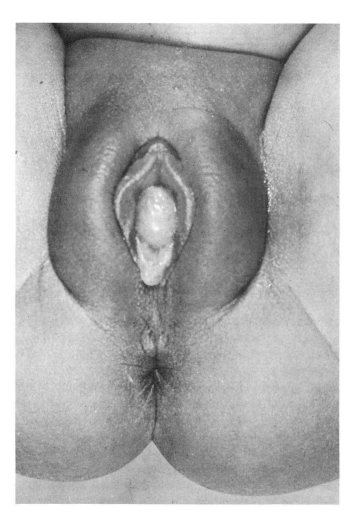

Fig. 3-41. Periurethral duct cyst bulging into anterior vaginal wall in a newborn.

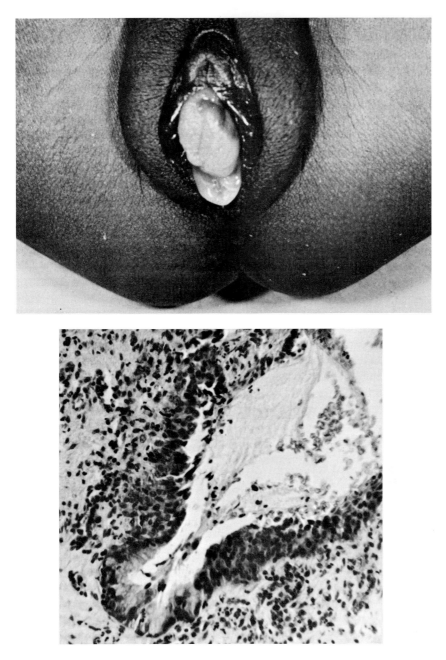

Fig. 3-42. Prolapse of anterior vaginal wall in newborn. *A*. Edematous hymen protrudes from labia posteriorly. Only abnormality of prolapsed vaginal wall was a mild inflammatory reaction. *B*. Photomicrograph of prolapsed vaginal wall. 240✕.

REFERENCES

1. BILL, A. H., JR., and JOHNSON, R. J. Failure of migration of the rectal opening as the cause for most cases of imperforate anus. *Surg Gynecol Obstet 106:*643, 1958.
2. BOLES, T. E., HARDACRE, J. M., and NEWTON, W. A., JR. Ovarian tumors and cysts in infants and children. *Arch Surg 83:*580, 1961.
3. BOWLES, H. E., and BURGESS, C. M. Apparent congenital absence of the uterus. *Am J Obstet Gynecol 38:*723, 1939.
4. CAMPBELL, M. *Clinical Pediatric Urology.* Philadelphia, Saunders, 1951.
5. CHATTERJEE, S. K., and TALUKDER, B. C. Double termination of the alimentary tract in female infants. *J Pediatr Surg 4:*237, 1969.
6. DUHAMEL, B. From the mermaid to anal imperforation: The syndrome of caudal regression. *Arch Dis Child 36:*152, 1961.
7. DUHAMEL, VON B., PAGES, R., and HAEGEL, P. Interpretationsversuch der anorectalen Missbildungen unter Bezugnahme einer neuer embryologischen Konzeption. *Z Kinderchir*, Suppl 1966, p. 83.
8. EDINGTON, G. H. Two unusual malformations of the hind end of the body. *Glasgow M J 96:*212, 1921.
9. EPPS, D. R., GUERIOS, M. F. M., NETO, A. S. C., LEON, N., and CINTRA, A. B. U. Clinical and microscopic findings in gonadal dysgenesis (Turner's syndrome). *J Clin Endocrinol Metab 18:*892, 1958.
10. EVANS, D. M. D., and HUGHES, H. Cysts in the vaginal wall. *J Obstet Gynaecol Br Commonw 68:*247, 1961.
11. FLORIAN, J. The early development of man, with special reference to the development of the mesoderm and cloacal membrane. *J Anat 67:*263, 1933.
12. GANS, S., and RUBIN, C. Apparent female infants with hernias and testes. *Am J Dis Child 104:*82, 1962.
13. HADDAD, H. M., and WILKINS, L. Congenital anomalies associated with gonadal aplasia. *Pediatrics 23:*885, 1959.
14. HAMILTON, G. M. Ovarian cysts in the newborn infant of diabetic mother. *J Obstet Gynaecol Br Emp 60:*533, 1953.
15. HENDRON, W. H., and CRAWFORD, J. D. Adrenogenital syndrome: The anatomy of the anomaly and its repair: Some new concepts. *J Pediatr Surg 4:*49, 1969.
16. HERTIG, A. T., and GORE, H. *Tumors of the Female Sex Organs.* Washington, Armed Forces Institute of Pathology, 1960, p. 79.
17. HUFFMAN, J. W. *The Gynecology of Childhood and Adolescence.* Philadelphia, Saunders, 1968, p. 329.
18. HUNG, W., and LOPRESTI, J. M. The high frequency of abnormal excretory urograms in young patients with gonadal dysplasia. *J Urol 98:*697, 1967.
19. JONES, H. W., JR., and HELLER, R. H. *Pediatric and Adolescent Gynecology.* Baltimore, Williams & Wilkins, 1966, p. 88.
20. KARRER, F. W., and SWENSON, S. A. Twisted ovarian cyst in a newborn infant. *Arch Surg 83:*921, 1961.
21. MAINOLFI, F. G., STANDIFORD, J. W., and HUBBARD, T. B., JR. Ruptured ovarian cyst in the newborn. *J Pediatr Surg 3:*612, 1968.
22. MARSHALL, J. R. Ovarian enlargement in the first year of life. *Ann Surg 161:*372, 1965.

23. MUECKE, E. C. The role of the cloacal membrane in exstrophy: The first successful experimental study. *J Urol 92:*659, 1964.
24. NICHOLS, D. H., and POSTLOFF, A. V. Congenital ectopic ovary. *Am J Obstet Gynecol 62:*195, 1951.
25. NOVAK, E. *Textbook of Gynecology,* 3rd ed. Baltimore, Williams & Wilkins, 1952.
26. PEGUM, J. M., LOLY, P. C. M., and FALKINER, N. McI. Development and classification of anorectal anomalies. *Arch Surg 89:*481, 1964.
27. POHLMAN, A. G. The development of the cloaca in human embryos. *Am J Anat 12:*1, 1911.
28. POTTER, E. L. *Pathology of the Fetus and the Newborn.* Chicago, Year Book, 1952.
29. RAVITCH, M. M. Hindgut duplication: Doubling of the colon and genital-urinary tract. *Ann Surg 137:*588, 1953.
30. RICHART, R. M., and BENIRSCHKE, K. Diagnosis of gonadal dysgenesis in newborn infants. *Obstet Gynecol 15:*621, 1960.
31. RICKHAM, P. P. Vesico-intestinal fissure. *Arch Dis Child 35:*97, 1960.
32. ROSS, L., and CARLSON, A. W. Incidental finding of an accessory ovary. *Am J Obstet Gynecol 100:*591, 1968.
33. SIEBER, W. K. Splenotesticular cord (splenogonadal fusion) associated with inguinal hernia. *J Pediatr Surg 4:*208, 1969.
34. SMITH, E. D. Duplication of the anus and genito-urinary tract. *Surgery 66:*909, 1969.
35. SOPER, R. T., and KILGER, K. Vesico-intestinal fissure. *J Urol 92:*490, 1964.
36. SPENCER, R., and LEVY, D. M. Hydrometrocolpos. *Ann Surg 155:*558, 1962.
37. SPENCER, R. Exstrophia splanchnica (exstrophy of the cloaca). *Surgery 57:*751, 1965.
38. SPENCER, R., and GEER, J. C. Ileo-cecal exstrophy with bifid intra-abdominal urinary bladder: Incomplete exstrophy of the cloaca. *J Pediatr Surg 2:*69, 1967.
39. TENCH, E. M. Development of the anus in the human embryo. *Am J Anat 59:*333, 1936.
40. WATSON, R. J. Splenogonadal fusion. *Surgery 63:*853, 1968.
41. WELCH, K. J. In Chapter 82. The female genital tract. In *Pediatric Surgery.* Mustard, W. T., Ravitch, M. M., Snyder, W. H., Jr., Welch, K. J., and Benson, C. D. (eds.). Vol. 2. Chicago, Year Book, 1969, p. 1382.
42. WHARTON, L. R. Two cases of supernumerary ovary and one of accessory ovary with an analysis of previously recorded cases. *Am J Obstet Gynecol 78:*1101, 1959.
43. WILLIS, R. A. *The Borderland of Embryology and Pathology.* London, Butterworth, 1962.
44. WOOLF, R. B., and ALLEN, W. M. Concomitant malformations: The frequent, simultaneous occurrence of congenital malformations of the reproductive and urinary tracts. *Obstet Gynecol 2:*236, 1953.
45. WYBURN, G. M. Development of infra-umbilical portion of abdominal wall, with remarks on aetiology of ectopia vesicae. *J Anat 71:*201, 1937.

Chapter Four

Congenital Adrenal Cortical Hyperplasia

Cary M. Dougherty

In a peculiar aberration of the natural development, hyperplasia of the adrenal cortex in utero causes that gland to produce an excessive amount of adrenal cortical hormone which, in turn, causes a masculinizing effect upon the genitalia of the female fetus. The hyperplasia and hyperfunction must be operative, of course, during the developmental stage when the external genitalia are not fully differentiated as female. The resulting effect is most startlingly apparent in the hermaphroditic appearance of the external sex organs. In addition, the masculinizing influence is evident later on in growth and development of the individual, when body contours and muscular development follow the male pattern. Nor are the morphologic abnormalities the only ones produced. Disturbances of metabolic processes related to and controlled by adrenal cortical secretions may be of such severity that they threaten the continued viability of the late fetus or newborn infant. Correction of the disturbed function often demands institution of measures remedial for the disturbed physiology first, before correction of anatomic mistakes due to the misdirected influence of the deranged endocrine gland.

EMBRYOLOGIC CONSIDERATIONS

The paired adrenals atop the kidneys are each composed of two separate glandular elements, cortical and medullary, having rather divergent function. Their development from two sources, one ectodermal and one mesodermal, initiates the dual purpose.

Cortex

The beginning of the adrenal cortex may be seen in the 8-mm, 5-week embryo. At this stage the longitudinal urogenital ridge is fully formed, with mesonephros occupying its lateral half and gonad the mesial portion. Mesodermal cells from the celomic epithelium and from the mesonephros push into the mesenchyme and form an elongated ovoid mass beneath the celomic epithelium at the root of the dorsal mesogastrium, extending along the cranial portion of the mesonephros from the sixth thoracic to the first lumbar segments. In this extensive area the primordium of the cortex is adjacent to and partly overlaps the gonad (Fig. 4-1). Because of the proximity of points of origin, as well as similarity of tissues of origin, the adrenal cortex and the gonadal stroma may be considered related organs.

Mesenchymal and mesothelial cells making up the adrenal cortical mass begin to take on characteristics which give them the appearance of "clear cells," a feature which may be seen in the cortical cells later to be derived from the early cells. Proliferation of these cortical cells continues at a rapid rate until soon the gland reaches a relatively enormous size. Its position is between the mesonephros and gonad laterally and the mesogastrium medially. Mesenchymal cells from the mesonephros ("Bowman's capsule") proliferate and surround the larger cortical cells to form the capsule of the gland.[7]

By the 14- to 16-mm, 6-week stage the cortex is invaded by neural components which initiate a different organization. Where originally the cortical anlage was an aggregation of differentiating elements, it is now composed of cells in masses and cords. During the eighth week, about 32-mm, there is extensive vascularization of the cortex with formation of venous sinuses dividing it into groups, clusters, and nests of cortical cells. The outer portion of the cortex arranged in this fashion constitutes the glomerular zone of the adrenal cortex. By the time the fetus reaches 44 mm, there are prominent cords arranged radially in the fetal fasciculoreticular zone. Further differentiation of the cortex does not take place in the fetus.

As soon as the fetal cortex is formed and organized, there is a second

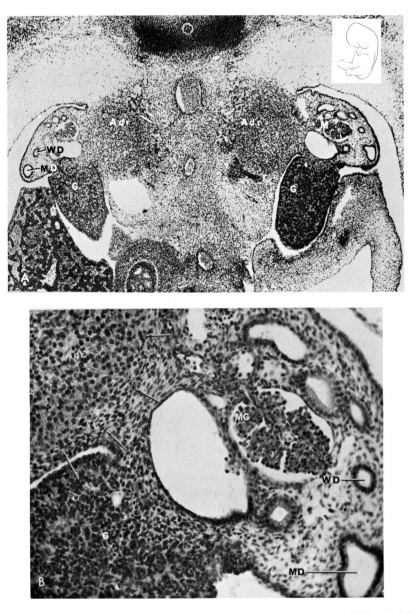

Fig. 4-1. Beginning development of adrenal cortex. Embryo 7707, 41-4-6; 14.5 mm, 5 weeks. *A*. Relation of ovary to adrenal. Fetal adrenal cortex (*Adr*) is formed medially and just dorsal to ovary (*G*) and medial to mesonephros (*M*) near cephalic pole of gonad. Adrenal grows to relatively great size. 45×. *B*. Fetal adrenal cortical cells (*Adr, arrows*) are in close relation to mesonephric glomeruli (*MG*), tubules, and duct (*WD*), müllerian duct (*MD*), and developing ovary (*G*). 200×. (Parts *A* and *B* from Dougherty, C. M. *Surgical Pathology of Gynecologic Disease*. New York, Harper & Row, 1968.)

wave of cortical cellular proliferation from the celomic epithelium and from dividing cortical cells already in place. This activity produces an enveloping mass of new cortex referred to as the *permanent* or *definitive cortex.* This change occurs about the 16-mm stage, somewhat earlier than a similar phenomenon in an adjacent site, that which builds the ovarian cortical stroma and secondary sex cords. The original cortical mass occupying all the central cortical region is the *fetal* or *provisional cortex,* while that portion resulting from the new proliferation is the permanent cortex.

At the time of birth the adrenal gland, made up mainly of the provisional cortex, is proportionately much larger than it is in later life (one-third the weight of the kidney at birth in comparison with one-twenty-eighth later).[2] Immediately after birth the provisional cortex begins a period of involution, with degeneration and dissolution of the provisional cortical cells chiefly in the fetal fasciculoreticular zone. Simultaneously there is replacement with cells of the permanent cortex, advancing from the glomerular zone. The change-over takes place within a few months after birth, but the subsequent organization of the adult type cortex is not completed until just before or about the time of adolescence. Thus, a normal or average schedule of histologic change in the adrenal cortex must be used to judge whether a gland is normal or abnormal at any given time in infancy or childhood.

Medulla

Details of the development of the medulla of the adrenal gland recognized today are those described by Zuckerkandl.[15] At about 4 weeks, 7 mm, certain undifferentiated neural elements of the paravertebral sympathetic ganglia medial to the adrenal cortical blastema migrate in the direction of the mass of fetal cortical cells. This phenomenon takes place from about the sixth thoracic to the first lumbar segments. The neural components consist of paraganglion or sympathicochromaffin cells and nerve fibers from the rami communicantes. Cells of the ganglia multiply by mitosis and the migrating cells start to invade the cortical cell mass from the medial side. Toward the thirty-fifth day, 14-mm stage, the paraganglion cells and neural tissue have pressed into the cortex to such an extent that they have appreciably increased the size of the gland. The complex of nerve tissue from which the neural elements are derived comprises mainly the celiac plexus, but it is also related to the superior mesenteric and renal plexuses. Migration of the paraganglion cells appears to follow the path of nerve fibers "scattered like seeds along the course of nerve tracts."[7] Continued cell multiplication is evident.

Chromaffin Cells

In the early phases there is no appreciable differentiation, but later, from about 30-mm stage, the paraganglion cells mature into chromaffin cells. Within the gland there is distribution of sympathetic nerves in the form of a plexus, similar to those of the periaortic plexuses. From this time on until the reorganization of the gland after birth, there is not a subdivision into cortex and medulla. Instead, chromaffin cells and sympathetic fibers are scattered throughout the cortex without definite organization. It is of interest to note that this is the same arrangement found in the adrenal gland of certain reptiles and adult birds.[13]

Differentiation of the paraganglion cells into chromaffin cells continues into the neonatal period. These cells accumulate the characteristic cytoplasmic pigment as the gland ages.

Double Origin

Because of its unique double origin and development, the adrenal gland is akin to two completely unrelated organs. The cortex arises close to, and its component cells possess some features in common with, the gonad, in particular, cells of the ovarian follicular theca and the testicular interstitial cells. The adrenal medulla is related to, and a part of, the chromaffin system including the carotid body and paraaortic bodies (organ of Zuckerkandl). It may be noted that the ovarian hilus cells seem to possess the same affinity for sympathetic nerves as that shown by the paraganglion cells, and under certain conditions hilus cells contain cytoplasmic pigment somewhat similar to that of adrenal chromaffin cells.

HISTOLOGY OF THE ADRENAL GLAND

Capsule

The thick, fibrous tissue capsule of the gland encases the cortex and sends trabeculae into the parenchyma. Sympathetic nerve fibers and small arteries penetrate the capsule and traverse the cortex radially from without inward, forming the sinusoids.

Cortex

Three layers of cortical cells not sharply demarcated from one another make up the larger part of the whole gland. These layers do not reach their final organization until the individual is several years or more of age. From the outer to inner the three are the *zona glomerulosa,* the *zona fasciculata,* and the *zona reticularis.*

Cells of the three layers have certain features in common. They are fairly large, they have a generous amount of cytoplasm which is stained pale with eosin or is even slightly basophilic, they have rounded vesicular or dark nuclei, and they more often than not contain cytoplasmic lipids. Cells of all three zones have been observed to divide by mitosis, apparently replenishing those elements which have been damaged or are in need of replacement.

In the *zona glomerulosa* the cortical cells are arranged in ovoid, round, or elongated groups separated by sinusoids or by a reticular network of connective tissue fibers. Cells are smaller than those of the other two zones, but cytoplasmic lipid material may be found.

Cells making up the *zona fasciculata* are appreciably larger and polyhedral, occurring in long cords. Bounded by the sinusoids of the vascular network, the cell cords are radially spaced and compose the major part of the cortex. Intracellular lipid is abundant. The cytoplasm of these cells especially is lightly stained and suggests the designation of clear cells.

In the *zona reticularis* the cells are little different from those of the fascicular zone. They are large, polyhedral, clear type, with cytoplasm which may be characterized as eosinophilic and smooth on section. There may be slightly less lipid material than is found in the midzone cells.

Medulla

The medulla is easily distinguished from the cortex when the adrenal gland is incised. The thick yellow cortical portion contrasts with the thin neutral-toned medullary part of the gland. In histologic sections the junction of the zona reticularis with medulla appears as an irregular but distinct line. Chromaffin cells are the dominant type found in the adrenal medulla. They are moderate sized to large and are arranged in random groups. Fixed in a solution containing potassium dichromate, their cytoplasm is seen to contain fine brown granules—the chromaffin reaction, a phenomenon brought about by the presence of epinephrine. Other large cells found in the medulla are the sympathetic ganglion cells, which are morphologically similar to the ganglion cells of the paravertebral ganglia. Scattered throughout the medulla are smaller, darker cells which are indistinguishable from, and probably are, small lymphocytes.

RELATION OF STRUCTURE AND FUNCTION

Corticosteroids

It is not yet well understood whether the different parts of the adrenal cortex manufacture different cortical hormones or whether there is a general synthesis of all hormones in the cortex as a whole. Certain experimental evidence supports the former hypothesis.[8-10] The principal functions of the adrenal cortex may be summarized as follows: maintenance of electrolyte and water balance through the operation of the *mineralocorticoids* (deoxycorticosterone and aldosterone); regulation of carbohydrate storage, mobilization, synthesis, and use through the activity of *glucocorticoids* (cortisone and hydrocortisone); and preservation of homeostasis of the connective tissues of the body, probably through one of the actions of cortisone. Studies appear to show that the zona glomerulosa is likely the site of production of mineralocorticoids, while the zona fasciculata elaborates glucocorticoids.

Sex Steroids

Both *androgenic* and *estrogenic* sex steroids are produced in the cortex of the adrenal gland. Except for urinary excretion of androgen metabolites during the first few weeks of postnatal life, there is no evidence of production of these hormones before the age of puberty. Adrenal androgens already identified are dehydroepiandrostenedione, androstenedione, and hydroxyandrostenedione. These are relatively weak-acting androgens compared with testosterone, but appear to be singularly active in promoting the growth of pubic, axillary, and body hair in the female. When they appear during the intrauterine period, these androgens effect masculinization of the external genitalia of the female and cause great enlargement of the phallus of the male fetus. They are responsible, along with the estrogenic hormones, for accelerated growth followed by epiphyseal closure in both sexes. Certain experimental evidence and pathologic observations indicate that the adrenal androgens are produced largely in the zona reticularis.[3, 11]

Histochemistry

Histochemical staining of sections of specially prepared and fixed gland tissue has, generally, not enabled investigators to identify the different hormonal substances in tissue sections. The use of several special stains together was at first thought to be specific for the 17-ketosteroids, but later this has been subject to some doubt.[4]

The adrenal medulla, unlike the cortex, produces and stores its two secretory products, epinephrine and norepinephrine (the catecholamines). These two hormones, stored within the cytoplasmic compartments of the medullary cells, are easily oxidized by the dichromate fixation and stained by ferric salts in reactions specific to the chromaffin system and adrenal medulla.

Abnormal Functions

Hyperfunction of the adrenal cortex may occur in the early embryo as a result of hyperplasia, or it may occur in the young due to neoplastic growth ("infant hercules"). Hypofunction is brought about by surgical removal or by destruction of the gland in disease, circumstances which lead to development of Addison's disease.

DEVELOPMENTAL STAGE AT WHICH ALTERATIONS APPEAR

It is possible to pinpoint the time at which, in embryonic development, the abnormal function of the adrenals begins to produce androgenic substances which act on the several target areas. This is the time at which the orderly development of the female genital organs is arrested and an abnormal state of masculinization begins to develop. The onset of the abnormal synthesis of steroids by the cortex is probably also the time when the adrenal begins its functions as a gland; it is probably not true that the gland first functions normally and then changes to an abnormal function. The targets, or end-organs, which reflect the influence of the abnormal androgenic cortical steroids are the genital tubercle in both sexes and the lower urogenital sinus in the female fetus. Assuming that the abnormal secretions would suppress the müllerian ductal structures and enhance growth of the wolffian duct and its derivatives, fetal development must have passed the stage at which ductal development and regression have occurred before adrenal cortical aberration takes place. It has not yet been proved that this represents the time of first appearance of increased secretion by the cortex, but that is the presumption. The following developmental landmarks are useful in determining the time of action of the androgens upon the female fetus:

1. Regression of the wolffian ducts is not interfered with, hence development has proceeded beyond the 60- to 75-mm stage.
2. Persistence of the pars phallica of the urogenital sinus is seen. This is a feature more nearly male than female, but the arrangement is seen in the 30- to 100-mm stage of female development.
3. Formation of the vaginal vestibule from the lower urogenital sinus is interfered with. The vestibule would have been evident by the 100- to 160-mm stage.
4. Fusion of the urethral folds, partially or completely, takes place. In the male the fusion to form the median raphe is complete about the 70- to 100-mm stage.

Thus the onset of function of the adrenal cortex in producing excess androgenic substances is about at the 60-mm stage, and not later than the 80-mm stage, of development of the female fetus.

PATHOGENESIS

Masculinization of the fetus, the hallmark of congenital adrenal hyperplasia, is brought about by presence of excessive amounts of adrenal androgenic substances. Excess production of these hormones is, in turn, a result of the malfunctioning of several enzyme systems within the cortex, specifically necessary for the biosynthesis of cortisol (hydrocortisone). The immediate effect is a failure of production of cortisol in the required amount. The lower level or the absence of cortisol signals the pituitary gland to secrete adrenocorticotropic hormone (ACTH) in greater quantity, whereupon this substance elicits both overgrowth of the adrenal glands and oversecretion of other cortical hormones the gland is capable of synthesizing.

There is yet another source of androgenic substances in the abnormal gland. While the manufacture of sufficient amount of cortisol is not possible, other enzymatic pathways proceed on an accelerated schedule under the influence of excess ACTH, producing an overabundance of other intermediate steroids and androgenic metabolites. These products, too, may exert virilizing powers.

Wilkins and others have identified defects in several different enzyme systems, all of which block synthesis of cortisol.[5, 6, 14] Depending upon which system is involved, the signs include simple virilization, virilization with hypertension, virilization with sodium ion loss, or incomplete virilization.

PATHOLOGIC CHANGES

The hyperplastic adrenal is greatly enlarged. The increased mass seems to be accounted for by a thickened cortex. The characteristic yellow color of the cortex is replaced by a paler yellow or white appearance, said to be due to absence of lipid material.

A number of observers have noted microscopically the increase in the proportion of cortex occupied by the zona reticularis.[1, 3, 11] The zona glomerulosa may not be recognizable as a separate entity or it may be essentially normal. Jones and Jones found hyperplasia of the zona glomerulosa in some instances.[12] The zona fasciculata occupies proportionately less space than in the normal gland. Lipid material may be decreased in the hyperplastic gland.

EFFECTS UPON THE MALE

The first signs of congenital adrenal hyperplasia in the male newborn may be those of salt-losing syndrome—vomiting, dehydration, and progressive pigmentation. The external genital organs may not show abnormality until months or years later. At that time there is progressive muscular and body development with enlargement of the penis and scrotum. The testes are small. After the initial acceleration of growth, premature epiphyseal closure takes place at a time when the individual is still shorter than the average for adults.

In some newborn males with congenital adrenal hyperplasia there is evidence of precocious development of the external genitalia (macrogenitosomia praecox) and pigmentation of the skin of the genital area. The penile enlargement is genuine, but the enlargement of the testes noted in some patients may be due to formation of large masses of adrenal-like cells believed by Wilkins to be aberrant adrenal tissue.[14] As a rule, the testes remain small and immature, and contain immature tubules as long as the excess androgenic state persists. Spermiogenesis does not occur as a rule, but may do so in the exceptional case.

Urinary excretion of ACTH is greatly elevated; 24-hour 17-ketosteroid determinations are high, but amenable to suppression by the administration of cortisone or dexamethasone.

In some forms of enzymatic defect causing adrenal cortical hyperplasia the patient may develop hypertension, believed due to prolonged effect of deoxycorticosterone.

EFFECTS UPON THE FEMALE

Urogenital Sinus

The earliest signs of masculinization of the female urogenital tract are related to the prevention of the transformation of the pars phallica of the urogenital sinus into the vaginal vestibule. The caudal portion of the sinus persists as a common passage connecting the urethra and the vagina with the external opening. This arrangement is more like that of the normal male, where the caudal part of the urogenital sinus is the common passage for urinary and genital tract secretions. Varying degrees of alteration may be found. Usually, there is one opening to the external surface, located at the base of the phallus, from which urine issues periodically. At a small distance inside the opening, the urethral orifice is visible. The vaginal opening should be at about the same level within the common passage and situated dorsal to the urethra. As this point represents the place where the vaginal vestibule ordinarily would be located, the examiner should be able to find a trace of the hymen at the vaginal opening. The hymen is much less prominent than when located in the normal position, but the mechanism of its formation, that of a transverse fold of sinus wall, would permit its development at the point of contact of the vaginal wall with the urogenital sinus. It is important to note that the hymen is not located at the opening of the urogenital sinus to the outside, i.e., at the base of the phallus.

It is equally important to note that the urethra does not open into the vagina or the vagina into the urethra. The illusions are due to the disproportionate sizes of the two tubular passages or to underdevelopment of the vagina.

In the less extreme forms of masculinization of the sinus, the urethral meatus may be identified in its usual location with the vaginal opening partly obscured by a high posterior fourchette. In these cases the abnormality of the urogenital sinus is very minor in extent.

In the more extreme virilization of the sinus, it may be hard to determine that the external genitalia were destined to be of the feminine gender. The pars phallica of the urogenital sinus may extend all the way to the tip of the clitoris as a phallic urethra. Except for its lack of a wide opening externally, the sinus is unchanged from its development in the 70-mm fetus, with vaginal and urethral openings at levels far within the common passageway.

External Genitalia

Virilizing congenital adrenal hyperplasia produces its most obvious effect in the enlargement of the clitoris. The enlargement may be so slight as scarcely to warrant the designation "abnormal" or so great as to suggest that the infant is male. A differentiating feature of some value is the greater amount of caudal angulation or curvature of the phallus seen in the female. The enlarged clitoris resembles the hypospadic penis with chordee. The glans clitoridis and the prepuce are prominent by virtue of being oversized, and these parts are generally the first noted to be abnormal.

The labia majora are altered by redundancy, wrinkling, and pigmentation of the skin. The labia minora are less conspicuous or partly blended with the large labia. In the severely virilized individual the labia are joined in the midline, forming a median raphe. The area of fusion may be partial or may extend the distance from perineum to phallus. When extensive, the resulting wrinkled, pouch-like structure is similar to scrotum in the cryptorchid male.

The external appearance and arrangement of the apertures of uro-genital sinus, urethra, and vagina may be confusing. If one recalls that the male penile urethra is actually a urogenital sinus and that the mas-culinized female system is similar to that of the normal male, the rela-tions of the altered female tract are better understood. In the mildly affected female, the external opening is slit-like and resembles the nor-mal vaginal vestibule, differing from the normal only in that it has a high posterior commissure. In other instances the urethral opening is visible, but that of the phallus is actually that of the urogenital sinus, while urethral and vaginal orifices are not exposed to view. The sinus aperture in the rare case is part way or all the way out on the phallus.

Somatic Changes

At birth the virilized female may not exhibit any abnormalities ex-cept those of the external genitalia. In some instances there may be pigmentation of the skin, particularly of the genital region, suggestive of the type found in Addison's disease.

In the untreated female beginning in early childhood gradual mascu-linization may be apparent in the development of body hair, facial hair necessitating shaving, and heavy musculature. At adolescence the breasts do not assume the female contour, but remain flat. The voice becomes coarser. There is a more rapid rate of growth in the early years, the child appearing taller than the normal for a given age, but premature closure of epiphyses of the long bones and cessation of growth produce a shorter than average adult.

The adolescent girl with unrecognized congenital adrenal hyperplasia experiences early signs of sexual maturity: pubic and axillary hair ap-pear, the growth spurt takes place earlier than expected; and growth ceases earlier than normal. Signs of ovarian function, however, never occur. The breasts are undeveloped and menstruation does not take place. The usual signs indicating ovulation are not evident.

Ovary

Jones and Jones described ovarian changes as those associated with suppression of a normal ovary and noted their reversibility when the suppressing cause is removed.[13] Follicle maturation does not occur, and ovulation and corpus luteum formation do not take place. The longer inhibition persists the more "aged" the ovary becomes. Primordial fol-licles gradually diminish in number and eventually disappear. Ovarian function with all its attendant signs usually begins upon the institution of proper treatment.

Uterus and Fallopian Tubes

The uterus and fallopian tubes are not affected in the fetus or new-born with adrenal cortical hyperplasia. Possible explanations for this are (1) a selective effect of the adrenal androgenic substance upon the genital tubercle only or (2) the commencement of operation of the androgenic effect at a time after the formation of these organs but before complete differentiation of the external genitalia.

Vagina

If the masculinization of the genital system of the female fetus does, indeed, begin rather late in its formation, aberrations of the vagina would be expected, since that organ is among the last to be completed embryologically. Such effects may be seen in the smaller and shorter size as well as the altered relation with the external opening. However, the tissues of the vagina may not be as reactive to the male hormonal effect since they are derived, not from the müllerian ductal system, but from urogenital sinus epithelial cells. The vagina may be only partially canalized, but this does not produce overt signs because adrenal hyperplasia suppresses menstrual function.

DIFFERENTIAL DIAGNOSIS

When *masculinization of the external genitalia* (pseudohermaphroditism) results from androgenic substance taken in or produced by maternal source, the individual has a karyotype of 46 XX, enlargement of the clitoris and labia, but no other stigmata. Urinary excretion of 17-ketosteroids is not elevated.

Masculinization caused by adrenal cortical tumor or, rarely, ovarian tumor, is essentially the same as that produced by adrenal cortical hyperplasia. Urinary excretion of 17-ketosteroids is elevated and is not suppressed by administration of cortisone or dexamethasone. A large adrenal tumor may be found upon examination, while a masculinizing ovarian tumor is sometimes palpable by rectal digital exploration.

Idiopathic sexual precocity or premature pubarche [15] produces early growth of genital and axillary hair along with other signs of sexual maturation. Urinary 17-ketosteroid excretion is not abnormal and genitalia are not hermaphroditic.

In *male pseudohermaphroditism* the male external genitalia resemble those of the masculinized female rather than those of the normal male. The chromosomal pattern of such persons is 46 XY, testes can be discovered, and urinary 17-ketosteroid excretion is not abnormal.

In none of the conditions to be differentiated from adrenal cortical hyperplasia is there a state of salt loss or of hypertension, as there may be with adrenal cortical hyperplasia.

A *male with cryptorchidism and hypospadias* may be mistaken for a female with masculinized external genitalia. Differentiation is based on the 46 XY karyotype, the finding of testes, the absence of vagina, cervix, and uterus, and the absence of abnormally high urinary 17-ketosteroid excretion.

Familial hirsutism sometimes suggests a mild degree of adrenal cortical hyperplasia. In most instances there are no demonstrable abnormal hormonal patterns, no elevation of urinary 17-ketosteroids, and no significant regression with a trial of therapy.

Masculinization associated with the *polycystic ovary syndrome* is not likely to be confused with adrenal cortical hyperplasia. The enlargement of the ovaries, the discovery of the disease sometime after the menarche, and the absence of abnormally high levels of urinary 17-ketosteroid excretion distinguish this entity.

Congenital adrenal cortical hyperplasia. CH64-76458. (Patient of Dr. Curtis Johnson, Louisiana State University School of Medicine, New Orleans.) This day-old infant was seen in consultation to determine whether it was male or female (Fig. 4-2). The consultant found upon questioning the mother that the child was the fourth offspring, that the mother had received no hormonal or other therapy during the pregnancy, that the delivery was uneventful. Among the siblings two brothers were living and well, while a sister had died at the age of 1 month. The sister had normal female external genitalia, however.

The consultant found the infant apparently healthy and normal except for malformed genitalia. The phallus was prominent and male-like, measuring 2.5 cm in length. The large labia looked more like scrotum, but no testes could be palpated within the redundant wrinkled sacs. There was a single opening at the base of the phallus through which urine was voided. Caudal to the opening the labioscrotal structures were joined in the midline. The pediatrician thought he was able to palpate the uterus by rectal digital examination.

Urinary 17-ketosteroid excretion was definitely elevated on two occasions: 1.06 mg/24 hours and 3.3 mg/24 hours (normal, less than 0.5 mg/24 hours). Sex chromatin was seen in cells of buccal smear. Electrolyte studies at intervals showed slight depression of the level of sodium, but no other major disturbances.

After a short initial period of observation during which the infant did not seem to do well, the pediatrician administered deoxycorticosterone acetate, cortisone, and a daily dietary supplement of salt.

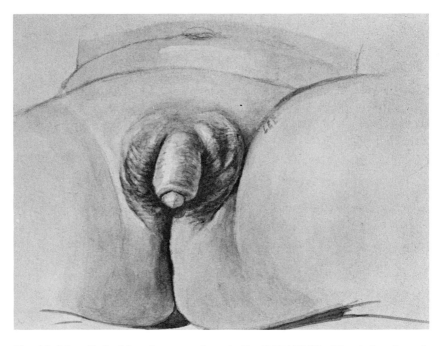

Fig. 4-2. Masculinized female external genitalia. CH64-76458. Clitoris is enlarged; labioscrotal folds are enlarged and skin is wrinkled and pigmented.

The patient improved and began to gain weight in a normal manner. At a later date corrective surgical operations were done upon the external genitalia to convert them to the female type. These procedures were removal of the clitoris and opening of the vaginal vestibule ("exteriorization" of the vagina).

REFERENCES

1. ANDERSON, W. A. D. *Pathology.* St. Louis, Mosby, 1966, p. 1118.
2. AREY, L. B. *Developmental Anatomy.* Philadelphia, Saunders, 1965, p. 519.
3. BLACKMAN, S. S., JR. Concerning the function and origin of the reticular zone of the adrenal cortex. *Bull Johns Hopkins Hosp 78:*180, 1946.
4. BLOOM, W., and FAWCETT, D. W. *A Textbook of Histology.* Philadelphia, Saunders, 1962, p. 365.
5. BONGIOVANNI, A. M., and EBERLEIN, W. R. Defective steroidal biogenesis in congenital adrenal hyperplasia. *Pediatrics 21:*661, 1958.
6. BONGIOVANNI, A. M. The adrenogenital syndrome with deficiency of 3-β-hydroxysteroid dehydrogenase. *J Clin Invest 41:*2086, 1962.
7. CROWDER, R. E. The development of the adrenal gland in man, with special

reference to origin and ultimate location of cell types and evidence in favor of the "cell migration" theory. *Contrib Embryol 36:*197, 1957.

8. GREEP, R. O., and DEANE, H. W. The cytology and cytochemistry of the adrenal cortex. *Ann NY Acad Sci 50:*596, 1949.

9. HECHTER, O., ZAFFARONI, A., JACOBSEN, R. P., LEVY, H., JEANLOZ, R. W., SCHENKER, V., and PINCUS, G. The Nature and the Biogenesis of the Adrenal Secretory Product. In Pincus, G. (ed.). *Recent Progress in Hormone Research,* vol. 6. New York, Academic Press, 1951, p. 215.

10. INGLE, D. Current status of adrenocortical research. *Am Sci 47:*413, 1959.

11. JONES, H. W., JR., and HELLER, R. H. *Pediatric and Adolescent Gynecology.* Baltimore, Williams & Wilkins, 1966, pp. 221, 222.

12. JONES, H. W., JR., and JONES, G. E. S. The gynecological aspects of adrenal hyperplasia and allied disorders. *Am J Obstet Gynecol 68:*1330, 1954.

13. NELSON, O. E. *Comparative Embryology of the Vertebrates.* New York, Blakiston, 1953.

14. WILKINS, L. *The Diagnosis and Treatment of Endocrine Disorders in Childhood and Adolescence.* Springfield, Ill., Thomas, 1965, pp. 401, 434.

15. ZUCKERKANDL, E. The development of the chromaffin organs and of the suprarenal bodies. In Keibel, F., and Mall, F. P. (eds.). *Manual of Human Embryology,* vol. 2. Philadelphia, Lippincott, 1912. Pp. 157–179.

Chapter Five

Anomalies of the Ovary and Testis

Cary M. Dougherty

The neutral or basic pattern in the mammalian species is the female. Mechanisms apparently exist in the very early development of mammalian and human embryos for the conversion of roughly half of the basic individuals to the modified model, the male type. Acceptance of this postulate is the key to understanding normal sexual differentiation. Certain of the specifics of the mode of operation of the process are not yet clear, but the underlying premise has been demonstrated in animal studies of normal and altered embryologic development. Clinical data offer additional support for the extrapolation of animal experimental findings to human sex differentiation.[1, 9] Sex differentiation, then, proceeds along the path of femaleness unless something happens to divert it to the path of maleness. Involved in this "something" are, chronologically, the chromosomes, certain hypothetical inductors, and the steroid sex hormones.

FACTORS IN DIFFERENTIATION OF THE SEXES

Defective development of the ovary or testis is manifested in the creation of abnormal forms or functions of one or more of the four major parts composing the embryologic, fetal, neonatal, and pubertal genital system. These subdivisions are (1) gonad, (2) ducts, (3) urogenital sinus, and (4) genital tubercle. Since the embryologic formation of the genital tract, like that of any other body system, follows the brick-on-brick method of construction, a malfunction of early development lays the foundation for a malformation of later-developing units of the system. An abnormality of development may begin at any time during the rather prolonged genesis of the genital system from early embryonic to late fetal periods. The organs involved in maldevelopment are those in the process of formation when the abnormal factor appears. In the embryologic time table the genital organs develop, with more or less overlap, in the order listed above. Thus, the normally formed or the malformed gonad is the first and essential brick upon which all later bricks are laid.

Chromosomes

The Y Chromosome

It is generally accepted that the human Y chromosome carries a gene (or genes) for the development of the testes. The single X chromosome probably does not carry a comparable or opposing factor for formation of ovaries. Rather, geneticists are of the opinion that the ovary develops in the absence of the Y chromosome.[1, 8] Further, evidence indicates that the Y chromosome is a very potent organizer, inducing formation of testes even when there are several X chromosomes in combination with the Y (Klinefelter's and "super" Klinefelter's syndromes).

There is at least one instance where a testis apparently develops in the absence of a Y chromosome, that is in true hermaphroditism, but this seems to be a single exception and may be explained on the basis that the Y chromosome is not absent but merely not detected, as in undiscovered mosaicism or inapparent translocation of a portion of the Y chromosome carrying the testis gene. A normal testis is probably never found in an individual without a Y chromosome. Conversely, when the chromosomal complement includes a Y, a testis of some sort is always formed.

Only one other trait is definitely attributable at this time to the Y chromosome in the human being—the trait for tall stature. The Y chromosome, or the testis, may prevent development of the stigmata of Turner's syndrome. However, this is at least in part hypothetical, because a second X chromosome also prevents the manifestation of the stigmata of Turner's syndrome.

The X Chromosome

The exact mechanism by which the X chromosome induces the formation of the ovary is not well understood. At least two conditions must be present: (1) there must be no Y chromosome, since in any combination of X's and Y's a testis, albeit not always functional, is always formed; and (2) there must be at least two X's. This suggests that if there is a trait on the X chromosome for formation of the ovary it must appear in both members of the pair in order to be effective.

Sex Linkage

Unlike the Y chromosome, the X carries many traits, both normal and abnormal.[21] The sex-linked disorders are among the factors so located. It should be noted that since most genes of the X chromosome are not paired with an allele on the Y, single recessive genes may manifest themselves in the male. This phenomenon cannot occur in the case of recessive genes on the autosomes where both members of the chromosome pair must carry the same recessive gene before the trait becomes manifest.

Sex Chromatin

In any individual with more than one X chromosome all but one of the X chromosomes are inactivated very early, possibly by the third week of embryonic development, in every cell. The inactivated X chromosome apparently undergoes condensation and assumes a position as a small chromatin bulge on the inner aspect of the nuclear membrane. Here it may be seen in the majority of the body cells, especially those with a normally vesicular nucleus. According to Lyon, the inactivation of the X chromosome in the normal female takes place independently (at random) and permanently in each cell.[20] If this hypothesis is correct every normal female is a genetic mosaic made up of approximately equal numbers of cells with inactivated maternal X and cells with inactivated paternal X. The two X chromosomes must exert a combined influence in the beginning, else the developing ovary would be like that of the X0 individual, a Turner's syndrome phenotype.

Polyploidy X, Y

Both X and Y chromosomes may occur in multiple numbers more readily than do the autosomes. Probably, ova with multiple sex chromosomes are more likely than normal ova to be aborted, but ova with multiple autosomes are even more likely to be nonviable or if viable, generally inferior.

Inductors

Embryologists believe substances exist which induce embryonic tissues to differentiate and produce special structures or organs. These substances are called inductors. They have certain peculiarities and modes of action which make them different from hormones, enzymes, or other secretions which operate continuously or intermittently. The inductor is active in one place and at one period of embryonic development. It is ineffective and probably not present at any other site and time. Most of our knowledge of inductors has come from experimental and comparative embryology, with relatively little but important information learned from observations of developmental errors in human specimens.

Testicular Inductor

In the human individual the Y chromosome appears to carry the testicular inductor. The time of its action is within the first 4 weeks of embryonic development, for during the fifth week its mark is evident when the indifferent gonad becomes recognizable as testis. Mesenchymal tissue from the urogenital ridge and mesonephros and epithelial cords from the celomic mesothelium make up the main portion of the emerging testis, the medullary portion of the undifferentiated gonad.

Ovarian Inductor

The mechanism by which the ovary is induced to differentiate from the indifferent gonad is not clear. Geneticists believe the X chromosome does not possess a gene comparable and opposite to the testis-inducing gene on the Y chromosome. Further, two X chromosomes must be present for the ovary to differentiate: Normal ovaries do not develop if the second X is either missing or deformed (X-ring, isochromosome X). An explanation, perhaps oversimplified, is that the ovary develops by the same mechanism as the somatic phenotype, i.e., in the absence of testicular inductor the indifferent gonad develops as an ovary.

Germ Cells as Inductors

It is a falsely appealing thought that the migrating germ cells of the indifferent gonad induce differentiation of the cortex in the case of the female germ cells and of the medulla in the case of the male germ cells. Such a theory would assume that if gonocytes with XY chromosomal content wandered into the gonad the medullary portion would develop, while if gonocytes with XX chromosomal complement arrived at the gonad cortical development would ensue. Such a theory would explain the development of both the normal and the dysgenetic gonad. A similar opinion has recently been expressed that the presence of germ cells in the gonad is a necessary condition for the development of the normal testis or ovary.[37]

Experimental studies have shown that this mechanism, whereby the germ cells act as inductors for the entire gonad, is operative in certain primitive animal forms, but it is not the mechanism of gonadal differentiation in mammals and man. In fact, the opposite condition probably prevails. The gonad or its cortex destined to be ovary induces the newly arriving germ cells to form oocytes, while the medulla or testis conditions the differentiation of spermatogonia.[16] Other experiments in mammals show that differentiation into testis or ovary takes place even if the germ-cell-bearing regions are destroyed before migration of the cells to the gonad.[16]

Another recent finding suggests that current ideas of the role of the germ cell in sexual differentiation must be revised. It has been assumed that in X0 individuals germ cells never reach the gonads.[12] Singh and Carr, however, found that the gonads of early embryos (up to a size of 23 mm, 6 weeks gestational age) with 45 X0 karyotype contained approximately the same number of germ cells as the gonads of similarly sized embryos with 46 XX (normal) karyotype. In older embryos the gonad in the abnormal type contained relatively more connective tissue and fewer germ cells than the gonad of the normal type.[29] This observation suggests that the gonocytes migrate into the gonad in the normal manner, but are lost at a later date by some unknown mechanism.[5] Hence, our presently held assumption that the gonad never possessed gonocytes is erroneous.

Maternal Hormones as Inductors

Also incorrect is the supposition that, in the absence of a fetal testicular substance, maternal *estrogens* are responsible for differentiation of the fetus as female. This would explain the finding that in the absence of testicular inductor the somatotype is female. However, in vitro experiments with rat embryos prove that the female differentiation takes place in the absence of maternal estrogen.[15] The maternal estrogen apparently influences fetal development only by its effect upon responsive fetal tissues such as vaginal epithelium. Maternal *gonadotropins* may play an indirect role in such activities as prostatic glandular stimulation in the male fetus or the estrogenic change in vaginal epithelium of the female. No evidence has been presented for function of either type of maternal hormone in the actual sex differentiation of the embryo.

Fetal "Hormones"

The *fetal testis* apparently produces a substance in utero which causes male differentiation of the wolffian duct and its derivatives, the urogenital sinus, and the genital tubercle and its structures. Though of undetermined nature, this substance is hormone-like in its action. Its effects may be partly reproduced by transplant experiments and by administration of the male sex steroids to the developing fetus, provided both procedures are started at an early enough stage of development.[16, 38]

There is undeniable morphologic evidence that the fetal testis both is acted upon and acts hormonally when in the fifth intrauterine month there is an overgrowth of testicular Leydig cells in the male gonad. Response of the interstitial cells to gonadotropin is a well-known phenomenon in the adult testis or even in the ovary. Whether these fetal Leydig cells produce appreciable quantities of male sex steroids is not certain, but such action may be presumed to occur at least on a small scale.

The *fetal ovaries* may produce hormone substances, too, although this action is not the counterpart of testicular function in the male. In the male, the wolffian ducts must be stimulated to develop. In the female, the müllerian duct develops in the absence of an inhibitory substance which would apparently be produced if there were a fetal testis, regardless of whether estrogen is present. Thus, an individual may have the normal female sex ductal structures even though "she" has no ovaries. Maturation of ovarian follicles is ample evidence of response of the late fetal ovary to gonadotropic hormone. Further, the maturing follicles probably produce estrogenic substances, at least in small amount.

These signs of hormonal activity of the fetal gonads last until near term in the male and until early postnatal life in the female, at which times the signs disappear.

Summary of Sex Differentiation

In the male zygote one or more genes probably located on the short arm of the Y chromosome initiate induction of male differentiation through testicle formation. When the embryonic gonad begins to develop medullary cords at 4–5 weeks, the action of the Y chromosomal inductor is probably concluded. Germ cells, recently arrived in the gonad from their primitive position in the entoderm of the yoke sac, align themselves in the medullary cords and are thereby induced to form spermatogonia. The fetal testis begins to elaborate (1) a substance which inhibits development of the müllerian duct and (2) a morphogenic substance which stimulates development of the male internal sex ducts from the wolffian ducts and male external genitalia from the genital tubercle. Hyperplasia of the interstitial cells starts midway in fetal development, and continued production of the fetal androgenic substance assures continued development of the male apparatus and its positioning in the proper somatic relations. Fetal interstitial cell hyperplasia subsides near the end of gestation when the testis enters its long latent period ending at puberty.

In the female zygote induction of femaleness is probably initiated by a gene or genes on the two X chromosomes, both members being a necessary and a sufficient inductor for ovary. Evidence is not so clear for this action in the case of the ovary-inducing genes as it is in that of the testis inductor. Differentiation of the gonad into ovary may be considered complete when the second wave of mesenchymal and celomic epithelial proliferation begins to displace the medullary cords as the main body of the gonad at 5–7 weeks. Germ cells arriving late and those already in the ovary settle in the new cortex and after proliferation are induced to become ovocytes. Germ cells remaining in the primary sex cords in the medullary portion of the ovary probably disappear along with the medullary cords by about the seventh month, 280 mm. In the absence of the müllerian inhibitor (elaborated only when a fetal testis is present), the müllerian ducts continue their evolution into the internal sex ducts of the female system. In the absence of the fetal morphogenic substance (produced only when a fetal testis is present), the wolffian ducts undergo involution, beginning at about the eighth week, 40 mm. In the absence of androgenic influence, the urogenital sinus and genital tubercle develop the form of femaleness. Probably in response to maternal or fetal gonadotropin, the ovarian cortex is organized in the familiar pattern, ovocytes surrounded by progranulosa cells and entering—but not completing—the first meiotic division. The process is completed near the seventh fetal month, at which time the ovary contains the peak number of germ cells, ovocytes. Shortly after the fetus emerges from the uterus most of the ovocytes and follicles undergo atresia and involution and the ovaries enter upon a prolonged period of inactivity awaiting maturation of the girl child.

DEFECTIVE OVARY SYNDROMES

Unilateral Ovarian Agenesis

In reviewing the records at Charity Hospital we found, among the intersex group, 6 case reports of unilateral absence of an ovary. The condition was not recognized every time by the doctor first treating the patient. Most of these patients displayed fundamentally different characteristics from those of the intersex group.

Ovaries

Among the 6 patients having only one ovary, 4 had the right organ and 2 the left. The lone ovary appeared to be in every way a normal organ. Where tissue was available for study, histologic sections showed normal follicular structures within a normal cortex. The absent ovary was not represented by a streak as is the dysgenetic gonad. Note was made of the absence of all supportive tissues in the region where the ovary should have been.

Tubes

The fallopian tube was absent on the same side where there was no ovary in each of the 6 cases.

Uterus

The uterus was unicornuate in 4, not examined in 1, and said to be normal in 1. The horn was on the side of the tube and ovary in the 4 patients, and all 4 uteri had the one round ligament on the side of the developed ovary.

On the side where the ovary was missing the uterus was described as being without attachments of any kind, including round ligament, broad ligament, and fallopian tube. That condition is typical of the unicornuate uterus even when there is an ovary present on the agenetic side. Uterosacral ligaments and lateral attachments of the cervix were the same as those found with the normal uterus.

In 1 patient the uterus was represented by unicornuate vestigial remnants. There was no endometrium. This patient also had agenesis of the vagina.

Vagina

A normal vagina was developed in 4 patients. In 1 the condition of the vagina was not described, and 1 patient had agenesis of the vagina (along with vestigial or rudimentary uterus).

External Genitalia

Detailed descriptions of the external genitalia were lacking. However, inasmuch as 4 of the patients ultimately gave birth to living children, the organs were at least functional if not cosmetically normal. In the patient with agenesis of the vagina, the labia and clitoris were said to appear normal.

One patient had masculinized female genitalia. The clitoris was enlarged to about 9 cm in length. Labia minora were not recognizable, but there was a median raphe where the vaginal opening was expected to be located.

Kidneys

Four patients having a unilateral ovary also had a unilateral kidney. In each, the single kidney was on the same side as the ovary. A fifth patient had two kidneys but one of the pair was located in the pelvic cavity, the normal one being on the side of the unilateral ovary. The sixth patient had two normally located kidneys.

Reproductive Record

Four of the six patients had living children. One patient died in infancy of congenital cystic disease of the lungs, thus precluding test of reproductivity.

Summary

Congenital absence (agenesis) of the ovary probably results from the unilateral destruction of a urogenital ridge, eliminating wolffian ductal derivatives as well as the fallopian tube and ovary on that side. The other ovary is not affected by the destructive process and retains its capability for function.

Absence of one ovary is not comparable to dysgenesis or abnormal development or to malformation of one or both gonads while they are in the indifferent stage of development. The only condition comparable to unilateral congenital absence of an ovary is absence of one testicle in the male.[4, 6]

Karyotypes and sex chromatin determinations were available on only 1 patient with unilateral ovarian agenesis. However, an individual capable of conceiving and carrying a pregnancy to term would in all probability have a chromosomal complement of 46 XX.

Congenital unilateral ovarian agenesis. CH62-19247. This Negro baby was thought to be a girl at birth. When the patient was 4 years old, a medical examination was done to establish the correct sex status. The clitoris was enlarged, the integument of the large labia was redundant and wrinkled, and the single opening was located at the base of the phallus. No labia minora were seen, but in their place was a median raphe. Laparotomy was performed for inspection of the internal genital organs. The left ovary and tube were completely normal. The right ovary and tube were nowhere to be found. The uterus was of the infantile type.

When she was 12 years old, she began having periodic bleeding. At the age of 18 years the patient was admitted to the hospital for revision of the external genitalia. The clitoris was amputated and the opening in the perineum (urogenital sinus) was enlarged. Vagina and hymen were inspected and found to be normal. Karyotype was 46 XX.

Several years later the patient became pregnant and was delivered of a living child. A second child was born 3 years later.

Turner's Syndrome (Gonadal Dysgenesis)

Definition

The definition of this disorder is the subject of considerable discussion. Originally referred to as ovarian agenesis or dysgenesis because affected individuals appeared female, the name was changed to gonadal dysgenesis when investigators found that the patients had a male sex chromatin pattern, i.e., no visible sex chromatin mass. The discovery that a missing sex chromosome was responsible for the male sex chromatin pattern did not simplify, but tended to complicate, terminology. It is now established that "females" having dysgenetic ovaries exhibit several different physical types as well as different assortments of sex chromosomes. Some of these physical stigmata may not be recognized at birth, the nature of the anomaly coming to light only later when the young woman does not begin to mature and to menstruate.

It is expedient at this time to define Turner's syndrome as a condition in which the gonads are represented by streaks of tissue resembling ovarian cortical stroma only, as distinguished from those conditions associated with aplastic or dysgenetic testes or ovotestes. Body types vary from normally feminine to severely stunted. Mental impairment may be associated.

Cause

The disorder is caused by abnormality of the sex chromosomes resulting in loss or destruction of all germ cells in the ovary and aplasia of the stroma.

Presenting Symptom

Short stature or amenorrhea at puberty prompt the patient to seek medical advice.

Gonads

The ovaries are best described as white streaks located in the pelvic region where the normal organs are found. They extend from the attachment of the utero-ovarian ligaments to a point near the lateral pelvic wall, joining the ovarian ligament there. The streak is 2–3 mm wide by about 4 cm long, suspended on the posterior (dorsal) leaf of the broad ligament by an ill-defined underdeveloped mesovarium. The appearance of the streak varies from barely noticeable to rather prominent. The stated dimensions also vary considerably. It is not unusual for one surgeon to state that the ovaries are absent in toto, while another notes later in the same patient that there are white streaks in the location where ovaries are usually found.

Although there are no visible follicles or follicular derivatives, there are sometimes nodules and yellowish-white masses in the dysgenetic ovary. Nodules of hilus cells or adrenal cortical cells are large enough to be seen.

The white streak may be shaped in a small rolled ridge, its color and texture suggesting a miniature ovary.

The dysgenetic ovarian streak is not positively identifiable by visual examination alone. One infant (Figs. 3-33 and 3-34) who appeared to have ovarian streaks actually had an exceptionally long thin organ which contained not only ova but a large follicle as well.

On histologic examination, a streak ovary exhibits enough character-istic features to be identifiable as ovary of a sort. There is a cortex con-sisting of fibrous tissue and modified fibrous tissue resembling the cor-tical stroma of the normal organ. Often this stromal tissue is identical in its morphologic and stain-absorbing properties with the normal ovar-ian stroma, and it occupies the same relation to the rudimentary organ as the cortical stroma does to the well-formed ovary.

A variety of structures usually thought of as belonging to the gonadal medulla may be seen in the streak ovary. The *wolffian duct* is often prominent. It is seen as the largest tubular structure in the sections of the gonadal hilum. Its columnar epithelium is similar to that of the fallopian tube but with smaller cells, while the circular, thin, muscular wall differentiates it from glandular elements. *Mesonephric tubules* (epoophoron) are usually numerous in the hilar region. These meso-nephric remnants as a rule do not undergo male-type differentiation. There is no suggestion of vas deferens or epididymis, although the per-sistent mesonephric tubules may suggest by their number an appearance of rudimentary epididymis. *Rete ovarii* is frequently prominent and identified by its irregular epithelium-lined spaces in the hilum. Since these vestiges are derivatives of the primary (medullary) sex cords, their prominence indicates more male-directed differentiation of the gonad than that seen in the normally differentiating ovary. *Hilus cells* (Leydig cells) are more numerous in the dysgenetic ovary than in the normal ovary. Often they may be seen in clusters and less often in small nodules several millimeters in diameter. In the dysgenetic ovary the hilus cells probably do not contain the cytoplasmic inclusions of Reinke.

Among the other structural features sometimes found are *adrenal cortical nodules,* the same morphologically as those seen in the normal ovarian hilum and in the kidney-adrenal areas. In one patient (CH58-280250) there were several adrenal cortical nodules in addition to sev-eral clusters of Leydig cells. At least one of the Leydig cell masses was considered as having characteristics of adenoma of those cells. One of the adrenal cortical nodules appeared to be made up of an inner core of Leydig cells and an outer cover of adrenal cortex. In this instance the Leydig cells did not possess the morphologic qualities of chromaffin cells of the adrenal medulla, although this resemblance has been pointed out a number of times.[10]

The hallmark of the dysgenetic ovary is the absence of follicular structures and ovocytes. Even though the appearance of the portions of cortical stroma suggests that additional sections might contain primordial follicles, these structures do not show up even on serial sections.

Fallopian Tubes and Uterus

The patient with Turner's syndrome usually has no developmental defects of the müllerian-derived organs. The tubes are described as thin, rudimentary, hypoplastic, or underdeveloped, but this appearance is only relative, for the tubes are completely formed and possess all the elements of the organ except maturity. They are comparable to the fallopian tubes of the prepubertal child, having a small fimbriated end, an ampullary portion, a thin isthmus, and a normal insertion into the cornual portion of the corpus uteri. In cross-section the villous folds of the tubal mucosa can easily be seen. The mesosalpinx is developed, and as in the normal female, may be seen to contain mesonephric remnants.

The uterus may be palpated in the central portion of the peritoneal fold forming the broad ligaments and mesosalpinx. Even though the uterus is small, it is in all other respects normal. Thin round ligaments attach at the right places on the corpus, and peritoneal folds of the uterosacral ligaments can be identified by tension. The small size has led to the false impression that the organ is vestigial and incapable of being induced to undergo maturation. Like the uterus of the infant and prepubertal child, the uterus of the female with Turner's syndrome is made up of a relatively large cervix and small corpus. The contrast in size of the two portions of the organ is a surprise to the surgeon who is more familiar with the proportions of the adult uterus and cervix.

On microscopic examination, the tubal epithelium resembles that of the unstimulated or atrophic organ. The uterine mucosa is similarly undeveloped, glands being relatively short simple tubes. Cervical columnar epithelium is further proliferated than either of the other two types. Glands are arranged in a compound formation.

Vulva, Vestibule, Vagina, and Portio Vaginalis of the Cervix

The external genitalia exhibit sexual infantilism, but in all other respects are normal. The mons veneris is almost devoid of pubic hair. The rounded, padded labia majora have little hair on their external surfaces and conceal by their prominence the clitoris and small labia. The labia minora are small, thin, and composed of pink mucosal folds. At their junction ventrally (anteriorly) they enclose the small glans clitoridis and corpora. If the labia minora are spread apart, the small but normally formed vaginal vestibule is visible. The urethral meatus is properly placed anteriorly to the vaginal opening with its hymen.

The vagina is regularly developed, its depth is often somewhat greater than would be anticipated on the basis of the immature appearance of the external genitalia. The hymen marks the junction of the vaginal opening with the vestibule, as in the normal female. Visualization of the vagina with a small self-illuminated anuscope or an air or water cystoscope proves that the rugous folds and mucosal walls are normal. The portio vaginalis of the cervix is inconspicuous, but when identified its shape is unmistakable. The cervical canal can be sounded with a fine probe.

A small minority of patients may exhibit a mild degree of masculinization of the external genital organs. In these patients there is more sexual hair and more growth and development of the labia majora and the clitoris. It is doubtful whether the masculinization associated with Turner's syndrome is ever sufficient to produce an actual phallus such as is seen in other types of intersex disorders. Masculinization in the patient with gonadal dysgenesis suggests another variant—asymmetrical or mixed gonadal dysgenesis.

Somatic Features

Dozens of characteristics have been noted in association with ovarian dysgenesis. Some of these are anomalies, but others are not considered to be such. The patient with ovarian agenesis may have a few, many, or none of the features noted. It could hardly be expected that one patient would possess all the anomalies described. Turner's original description comprises three features externally visible: infantilism, webbed neck, and cubitus valgus.[36] Other characteristics are puerile breasts, receding chin, brachycephaly, low-set ears, high-arched palate, pigmented nevi, urinary tract anomalies, color blindness, short neck, low hair line, aging of skin, short stature, shield-shaped chest, coarctation of the aorta, cardiac septal defects, and aortic stenosis.

Hormonal Pattern

Estrogenic effect on receptive tissues is very slight, and assay of these steroids reveals very low levels. Androgenic hormones and 17-ketosteroids are also very low. The most important endocrinologic finding is elevation of pituitary gonadotropin (follicle-stimulating hormone, FSH) to a level within the range of menopausal values. A few individuals with gonadal dysgenesis do not have elevated FSH values, but these are the exceptions.

Chromosomal Patterns

Cells collected from most of these patients and examined are seen to have no nuclear sex chromatin mass. The karyotype shows that one sex chromosome is missing—the pattern described as 45 X0. The remaining sex chromosome is always an X. Patients having this arrangement of chromosomes generally present the whole picture of Turner's syndrome with assorted localized anomalies.

A second pattern is a full complement of chromosomes but an abnormally formed X. The abnormality is caused by deletion of part of one X, by ring formation, or by "isochromosome" formation. The karyotype is designated as 46 X deleted-X or 46 X iso-X. Patients with this chromosomal pattern have cell nuclei with sex chromatin mass.[8]

A third chromosomal pattern is the mosaic pattern. Some of the body cells and their progeny exhibit one pattern, e.g., 46 XX, while other body cells and their progeny show a different pattern, e.g., 45 X0. The observed mosaic patterns are X0/XX, X0/XXX, X0/X iso-X, and X0/X deleted-X. Other chromosomal patterns have been described in a few instances and await verification by additional studies.

Variation in Somatotypes

Patients with Turner's syndrome show a number of different somatotypes. The constant feature is the presence of streak or aplastic gonads. The range of somatotypes extends from the extremely abnormal female of short stature to the female who apparently is completely normal. The patient with dysgenetic gonads and normal somatotype has been referred to as having "pure gonadal dysgenesis."

An occasional patient may have hypertrophy of the clitoris. This finding may be, but usually is not, associated with other evidence of masculinization. This effect is the result of action of one of the androgenic substances, but which one has not been determined.

There is no rule regarding the number and kinds of defects in any one individual. Patients having an X0 pattern or mosaicism including an X0 stem may tend to have more localized anomalies than others.[8]

Treatment

Almost all medical authors recommend that patients suspected of having dysgenetic gonads undergo laparotomy as the final step in the diagnostic study. The only definitive procedure need be the removal of the gonadal streaks, together with their mesenteries. The infantile tubes and uterus can be stimulated by exogenous estrogen.

Oral estrogen should be given in graduated dosage starting at about the time the patient would ordinarily begin sexual maturation. The initial dose should be about 1.25 mg of conjugated estrogens daily for 25 days each month. For the average girl this dose is increased to 2.5 mg daily after 2 or 3 months. Within 3 months this dose of estrogen usually stimulates growth of the uterus and endometrium with production of a menstrual flow. After a number of cycles of treatment with estrogens, the patient may experience prolonged or profuse menstrual bleeding or intermittent episodes of spotting and bleeding. When this irregularity develops, a progestational substance should be given which causes ripening and self-limited shedding of the endometrium in the withdrawal intervals.

Estrogen substitution therapy should probably be considered as permanent treatment. The necessary safeguards must be outlined to the patient and instituted as routines. These include periodic vaginal and cervical cytologic smear, curettage of the endometrium in the event of irregularity in bleeding, careful breast examinations, and pelvic examinations.

Turner's syndrome. CH68-195242. This 43-year-old Caucasian female was seen by a neurologist because she thought she was losing her memory. Prolonged questioning of the patient and her husband led the neurologist to believe she was mentally below average. Married and childless a number of years, the couple had never had complete sexual intercourse.

Examination by an endocrinologic consultant showed the following abnormalities: short stature (52 in.), infantile but otherwise normal external genitalia, sparse pubic and axillary hair, and cubitus valgus. Other stigmata noted were amenorrhea, lack of breast development with infantile areolae and nipples, and many pigmented nevi over the body. Pelvic examination confirmed the finding of infantile but normal genitalia. The uterus was palpated. The patient refused surgical operation for inspection of internal genital organs.

Cells of buccal smears did not possess sex chromatin, and chromosomal complement was 45 X0 (Fig. 5-1). Pituitary FSH level was high. Vaginal cytologic smear reflected low estrogenic activity.

When given moderate doses of estrogen orally in cycles, the patient began having vaginal bleeding.

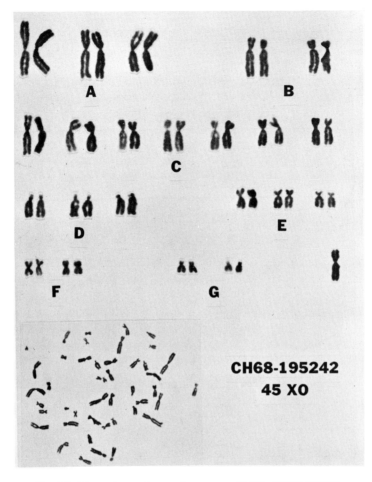

Fig. 5-1. Turner's syndrome, karyotype 45 X0. CH68-195242.

Gonadal agenesis with vaginal agenesis and 46 XY karyotype. CH63-40995. A 16-year-old Negro consulted the clinic gynecologist because she had not menstruated. Examination disclosed that she was of small stature, had puerile breasts and nipples, and had no axillary or pubic hair. The external genital organs were infantile, with small labia and clitoris. There was no vaginal opening, and the examiner thought of "imperforate hymen."

Intravenous pyelography demonstrated normal kidneys and ureters. Urinary excretion of pituitary FSH was elevated (104 MU/24 hours), but 17-ketosteroid level was normal (7.4 mg/24 hours). Somatic cells did not contain sex chromatin, and the chromosomal complement was 46 XY (Fig. 5-2).

At laparotomy the surgeon could not identify any internal genital organs. Tissues removed from the areas where the organs should have been were reported by the pathologist as being fibrovascular tags. Inguinal canals were examined and found not to conceal gonads.

When the suspected imperforate hymen proved to be vaginal agenesis, an artificial vagina was constructed. Estrogen substitution treatment was begun.[7]

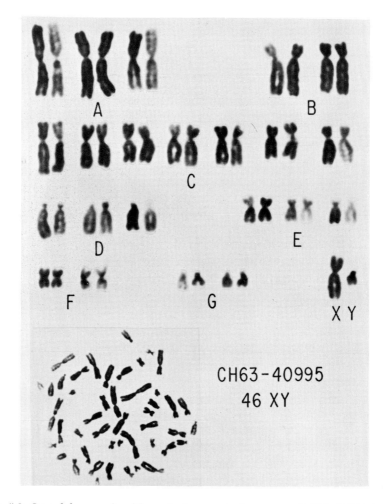

Fig. 5-2. Gonadal agenesis with vaginal agenesis, karyotype 46 XY. CH63-40995.

DEFECTIVE TESTIS SYNDROMES

Mixed Gonadal Dysgenesis

Definition

On the basis of the morphologic characteristics of the gonads, mixed gonadal dysgenesis may be defined as a condition in which there are any two of three types of gonads: a testis, a streak, or a gonadal tumor (of the germ cell or sex cord types).[8, 31] Although some authors do not segregate the entity,[27] this syndrome differs fundamentally from Turner's syndrome. The gonads in Turner's syndrome are either bilateral streaks whose appearance suggests ovarian cortical stroma or, rarely, hypoplastic ovaries; in mixed gonadal dysgenesis male elements are distinguishable in both gonads. Hence there is ground for speculation that the individual with Turner's syndrome may be fundamentally different from the person with mixed gonadal dysgenesis.

Gonad

In the individual whose gonads are testis and streak the testis is usually recognizable at the time of operation by its smooth, white tunica. The testis may be located at any point along the pathway of migration from pelvis or pelvic brim to inguinal canal, but is often intraabdominal in the location where the ovary would be ordinarily.

On histologic examination the testis is seen to be severely dysgenetic. Primary medullary tubules are composed of Sertoli-like or undifferentiated cells. Leydig interstitial cells are overabundant in the fibrous stroma. Germ cells (spermatogonia) are not usually found.

The streak gonad in mixed gonadal dysgenesis contains three elements of the male gonad: imperfect primary sex cords or tubules (seminiferous tubules), Leydig cells, and more or less prominent remnants of the wolffian body and duct.

Fallopian Tubes and Uterus

When the testicles or gonads are severely dysgenetic, the sex ducts develop along female lines, apparently in keeping with Jost's hypothesis. At laparotomy the internal organs are usually found to be similar to those described in Turner's syndrome, i.e., normally female but of the immature or prepubertal type.

External Genitalia

The clitoris is enlarged, often to a marked degree, forming a penis-like phallus. The vaginal vestibule is modified by fusion of the labia minora to some extent. A persistent urogenital sinus is present if the fusion is nearly complete. A small common tract opens at the base of the phallus. In short, the external genital organs appear to be masculinized female type.

Somatic Types

Individuals having mixed gonadal dysgenesis may show the triad of anomalies characteristic of Turner's syndrome: infantilism, webbed neck, and cubitus valgus. Some individuals look like normal females, while others show signs of masculinization.

Hormonal Pattern

The significant abnormality is the same as that found in Turner's syndrome: an elevated FSH value near the level of that hormone found in the postmenopausal female. The 17-ketosteroids and generally other androgenic substances are present at about the normal levels for females. Somewhat higher amounts of these hormones may be noted in the individual with external signs of masculinization.

Chromosomal Patterns

In the few well-studied patients, the chromosomal complement seems to be mosaic. The pattern is most likely to be an X0 stem with another stem containing a Y. In the case reports summarized by Federman the pattern found most often was X0/XY.[8]

Gonadal Tumors

Women with this type of gonadal dysgenesis appear to have a strong predilection for developing tumors. However, the definition incorporates a built-in bias because all patients with gonadal dysgenesis with a tumor on one side are classified as having "mixed" gonadal dysgenesis. The tumors are usually of the type involving germ cells—a paradox, since the dysgenetic streak gonad usually contains no germ cells.

A pathologically interesting tumor involving the dysgenetic streak is the *gonadoblastoma*,[25, 28] or gonocytoma.[35] The gonadoblastoma forms a small mass in the dysgenetic gonad or replaces it completely. Microscopic sections show germ cells (gonocytes or spermatogonia), follicular-tubular elements (Sertoli-granulosa cells), and stromal components (Leydig-theca cells). The architectural arrangement of these diverse components is reminiscent of that of granulosa–theca cell tumors and seminoma-germinoma tumors. Laminated calcific concretions are a common feature of the gonadoblastoma. Some authors believe the gonadoblastoma is a product of the dysgenetic gonad exclusively.[22]

Treatment

In mixed gonadal dysgenesis the need for laparotomy is urgent because of the possibility of gonadal tumors. Estrogen substitution is indicated in these patients, but not unless the dysgenetic gonads have been surgically removed.

Individuals with mixed gonadal dysgenesis may have external genitalia of the masculinized female type. In all cases, possibly excepting the most strongly masculinized, the external genitalia should be revised surgically to function as female. In most instances this revision means amputation of the phallus, reconstruction of the vaginal vestibule by opening fused labia minora and a part of the perineal body, and reestablishing the opening of the vagina in its normal relation to the vestibule and the exterior aperture of the pudendal area ("exteriorization" of the vagina).[14]

Mixed gonadal dysgenesis versus male pseudohermaphroditism. BR-702008. (Patient of Dr. Douglas Gordon, Baton Rouge.) This white female patient was seen by Dr. Gordon when she was 13 years old. She was less mature than her classmates and had not begun menstruation. The parent stated that the child had been born with ambiguous genitalia which looked more like female than male organs. At the age of 2 years a surgical operation upon the external genitalia removed the phallus and enlarged the vaginal opening; laparotomy was included. The surgeon described a right testis and epididymis, vas deferens, fallopian tube, a uterus, and a left ovary with fallopian tube. He removed the right gonad (testis), the epididymis, and the vas. The left gonad he thought to be a grossly normal ovary and accordingly he did not secure a tissue specimen.

At the age of 13 years, the patient's height was average for an 11-year-old female and her facial and body characteristics were commensurate with that chronologic age. There was no breast maturation and no appreciable axillary or pubic hair growth. The body proportions suggested the eunuchoid pattern.

The clitoris was absent. The labia, vestibule, hymen, vagina, and portio vaginalis of the cervix were all of the infantile type but otherwise essentially normal.

Hormonal assay showed pituitary gonadotropin FSH, 50–100 MU (elevated); total estrogens, 9 μg/24 hours (slightly low); 17-ketosteroids, 6.9 mg/24 hours; 17-ketogenic steroids, 6.1 mg/24 hours (normal female). A buccal smear was thought to show male pattern, i.e., no sex chromatin. Karyotype was 46 XY, determined by counts of 85 cells and typing of 11 photographs of cells (Fig. 5-3).

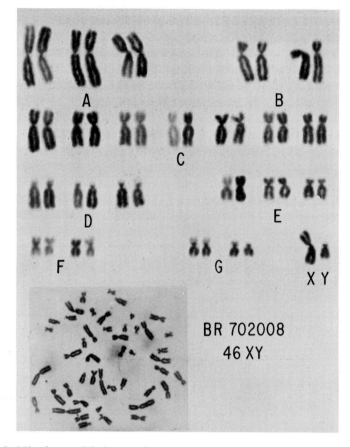

Fig. 5-3. Mixed gonadal dysgenesis versus male pseudohermaphroditism, karyotype 46 XY. BR-702008.

Microscopic examination of the right testis showed an immature
and dysgenetic gonad (Fig. 5-4*A–D*). It was composed of fetal-type seminiferous tubules having a thickened and hyalinized basement membrane. Cells lining the tubules appeared to be immature or undifferentiated Sertoli cells with a few larger, clear cells resembling spermatogonia. In a few tubules there was more advanced degeneration
with deposition of small calcific bodies. No tubule had a lumen and
there was, of course, no maturation of germ cells. There were a few
interstitial cells between the tubules, mostly spindle-shaped.

The patient and her mother declined the recommendation of the
gynecologist for a second laparotomy.

The consultants were of the opinion that if the remaining gonad

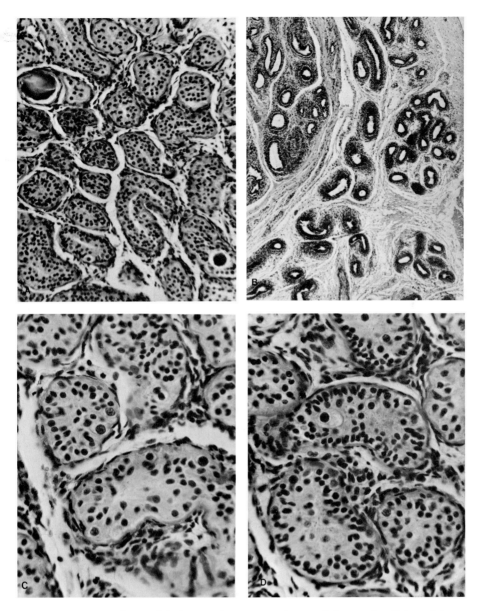

Fig. 5-4. Mixed gonadal dysgenesis versus male pseudohermaphroditism. BR-702008. *A*. Right gonad showing fetal-type seminiferous tubules. Tubules have no lumina. Two calcium bodies may be seen within tubules. 240×. *B*. Tubules found in hilum of gonad probably represent epididymis. 70×. *C*. Cross-section of seminiferous tubules show predominant cells to be undifferentiated type. Occasional larger clear cells may be spermatogonia. 480×. *D*. Occasional large clear cell stands out among surrounding undifferentiated tubule cells. Interstitial cells may be seen between seminiferous tubules, although not in great numbers. 480×.

were, indeed, an ovary or ovotestis, it was probably not functioning as indicated by the high FSH value. On the other hand, the left gonad might be a dysgenetic gonad or streak instead of an ovary. If ovary or ovotestis were present, the condition would be true hermaphroditism, while if a dysgenetic streak gonad were discovered at a second laparotomy, it would be mixed gonadal dysgenesis. If the remaining gonad were another testis, the condition would be male pseudohermaphroditism with phallic enlargement and partial masculinization of the external genitalia. In any of these cases, since the patient has reached puberty, the functionless dysgenetic gonad should be removed and estrogen substitution initiated.

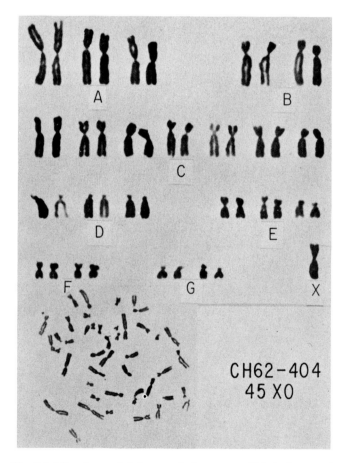

Fig. 5-5. Mixed gonadal dysgenesis, karyotype 45 X0. CH62-404.

Two important points are illustrated by this case. First, laparotomy is diagnostic as well as therapeutic, and therefore specimens from both gonads must be examined histologically. Second, there may be very few differences visible on external examination among these three types of intersex persons.

Mixed gonadal dysgenesis. CH62-404. A 22-month-old Negro was examined by a pediatrician and found to have enlargement of the clitoris along with otherwise unremarkable infantile genitalia. Electrolyte and hormone excretion studies were all normal. Nuclei of buccal smear contained no sex chromatin. The karyotype was a mosaic pattern, 45 X0/46 XY (Figs. 5-5 and 5-6). These two patterns were the only major stems seen on several different cultures of lymphocytes.

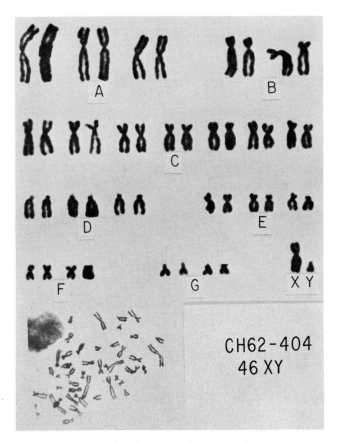

Fig. 5-6. Mixed gonadal dysgenesis, karyotype 46 XY. CH62-404.

At laparotomy the surgeon identified a right gonad measuring 1.5 by 1.5 cm, a right fallopian tube, a left gonadal streak, and a left fallopian tube. The uterus was normal. Gonads and ducts were removed surgically.

Histologic examination showed the right gonad to be made up principally of immature seminiferous tubules. A smaller part was fibrous-like ovarian cortex. The immature testicular tubules contained only undifferentiated cells suggestive of Sertoli cells. A few tubules contained calcific bodies with concentric rings of calcium. There were very few interstitial cells. In the stromal portion a single primordial follicle containing an ovum was seen. In addition to the right fallopian tube there were a right vas deferens, epididymis, and rete testis. The left gonad was made up of a connective tissue stroma resembling ovary. No ova were seen.

First classified as a true hermaphrodite, this patient manifested more characteristics of mixed gonadal dysgenesis. After amputation of the clitoris, she was reared as a girl.[7]

Testicular Feminization (Morris' Syndrome)

Definition

Testicular feminization is defined by its characteristics, listed by Morris as follows:

"1. Female habitus. In some cases the build has a eunuchoid tendency.

"2. Normal female breasts, often with tendency to be 'overdeveloped,' although the nipples are sometimes juvenile.

"3. Absent or scanty axillary and pubic hair in the majority of cases. There may be a slight amount of vulvar hair. The hair on the head is that of a normal female without temporal recession, but the facial hair is more often absent, as in a child.

"4. Female external genitals. The labia may be underdeveloped (infantile or puerile), especially the labia minora. The clitoris is normal or small. The vagina ends blindly, but is usually adequate for marital relations.

"5. Absence of internal genitals except for rudimentary uterine and other anlage, including sometimes fallopian tubes or spermatic ducts, and for the gonads, which may be intraabdominal or may lie along the course of the inguinal canal.

"6. Gonads consisting largely of seminiferous tubules usually without spermatogenesis, but in most cases with a marked increase in interstitial cells. The picture is essentially that encountered in cases of undescended testes. Tubular adenomas are frequent findings. In a

few cases there has been a considerable amount of fibrous stroma.
"7. Hormone assays in a limited number of cases suggest that these testes produce both estrogen and androgen. The pituitary gonadotropins have been elevated in some instances." [23]

The individual with testicular feminization, then, is one whose only internal genital organs are ectopic testes, but whose external appearance and genitalia are those of a normal female.

Cause

Probably a heritable defect is responsible for production of testes with completely inadequate function. Testosterone insensitivity may be a causal factor.

Presenting Symptom

Amenorrhea at puberty is the first indication of abnormality.

Testes

The smooth, white testes are easily distinguished from ovaries. At one pole of the organ, the one which may be thought of as the advancing pole, there is a conical epididymis or connective tissue accumulation where the gubernaculum testis is attached. The testes are usually, but not invariably, ectopic. When ectopic they are in the inguinal canal, suspended from the region of the internal inguinal ring, or even positioned where ovaries would be found. Usually the gubernaculum may be identified at the forward pole. A prominent feature is the thick, smooth, white tunica vaginalis testis. When the tunica is incised, the mass of the seminiferous tubules appears as mushy brownish-yellow interior of the testis. Adenomas, when large enough, may be palpated, but this step is not reliable to rule out the presence of small tumors or of nodular hyperplasia.

Using microscopic and ultramicroscopic means a number of authors have been able to specifically characterize the testis of testicular feminization,[10, 24, 26] although at least one is of the opinion that there is no characteristic histologic picture.[11] The tunic may be more fibrotic than that of a normal testis, but it is otherwise not remarkable. Seminiferous tubules are of the immature type, not patent but with a lining of "primitive germ cells" or undifferentiated cells suggestive of spermatogonia.[19] For the most part there is no evidence of germ cell activity or spermatogenesis, but the phenomenon has been observed and presence of sperm has been reported.[39] Sertoli cells, possibly not of the exact type found in the normal testis, have been seen. The number of Sertoli cells is relatively small, and in some specimens none may be discernible.

Two signs indicate that the testis is dysgenetic: (1) there may be small calcium concretions within seminiferous tubules, of the type found in certain gonadal tumors, and (2) the sheaths of the tubules may be thickened or even hyalinized (occasionally the entire structure of seminiferous tubules has undergone hyalinization, forming ghost tubules).

Interstitial cells, by comparison with the normal testis, are more numerous than expected. Both immature and mature types may be found. The distribution of these elements is somewhat different, too. Relatively few are found between tubules, but instead the interstitial tissue is more fibrous. In the septa near the capsule and in the testicular hilar regions are large aggregations of interstitial cells, some of which possess the typical appearance of mature Leydig cells. Within the clear or light cytoplasm are fine granules of brown-stained material, said to be indicative of secretory activity. Several authors have reported seeing crystalloids of Reinke in a few cells. The rounded, vesicular nuclei are easily seen to have no sex chromatin mass, the expected male pattern.

Internal Genital Organs

Other internal genital ductal derivatives are rudimentary or absent. Fallopian tubes and uterus, the products of müllerian differentiation, are represented by thin condensations of fibromuscular tissue within a curved transverse fold of peritoneum stretched between the two gonads. Vas deferens and epididymis, the progeny of wolffian differentiation, are usually rudimentary. In some cases the testis is surmounted by a conical mass of fibroepithelial tissue, variously described as uterine horn, prostatic remnant, epididymis, or gubernaculum testis.

External Genitalia

An exceptional characteristic immediately obvious is the absence of sexual hair. Since this is the only external difference and since prepubertal girls do not possess such hair, there may not be any distinguishing external features in early childhood. An equally important sign is the finding of a short or shallow vagina which does not connect internally with a cervix uteri. The vagina is small but its lining is rugous, comparable to the vaginal lining of similarly aged normal females.

Labia majora, labia minora, clitoris, urethral meatus, vaginal vestibule, and hymen are all completely normal except that there is no vulvar hair. The state of development may be infantile or puerile.

Somatic Features

The individual with testicular feminization possesses, essentially, a completely feminine body without sexual and axillary hair. Medical authors almost without exception use superlatives in referring to excellence of breast development and feminine contours. Among the finer points of difference between this female and her normal sister is a tendency for more puerile breast nipples and areolas. Inguinal hernia, unilateral or bilateral, is common.

Hormonal Patterns

Hormonal characteristics of testicular feminization are not fully known. The following summary represents a consensus among endocrinologists. *Estrogen* determinations are slightly lower than those found in the normal female adult and slightly higher than those of the adult male. No qualitative difference between normal and affected individuals has been discovered. *Androgen* levels are somewhat lower than those of the unaffected male but no demonstrable qualitative difference has been consistently found. *Gonadotropin* values have been reported as higher than normal and as about normal. Removal of the feminizing testis causes a rise in gonadotropin level, comparable to that of the postmenopausal female. Withdrawal of the endogenous estrogen supply by orchiectomy results in onset of hot flushes.

Chromosomal Pattern

The only pattern for this type of intersex is the normal male pattern, XY. Cells of the buccal smear do not have a sex chromatin mass.

Variations in Somatotypes

There is much less variation in individuals with testicular feminization than in the other types of gonadal dysgenesis. However, some of these females have a degree of masculinization of the external genitalia, while others may possess a uterus. These are not in the strict sense instances of testicular feminization, but their existence proves once again that there is a continuum of sexual differentiation from the completely feminizing, nonmasculinizing testis to the normal masculinizing testis.

Inheritance

Testicular feminization occurs in families. The affected female members carry the traits and seem to transmit the abnormality to about half the male offspring of the carrier mother. The recognition of the fact of inheritance is reflected in the name given to this condition by medical authors, familial male pseudohermaphroditism. Geneticists now believe that the manner of inheritance is either as an autosomal dominant expressed only in the male or as a sex-linked recessive characteristic.[8, 10] Exactly what is inherited is not clear. If it is a trait for a testis with defective enzymatic pathways, as one author believes, the gene would be on the Y chromosome.[10] If it is a trait for defective end-organs, possibly an autosome is involved.[11]

Treatment

After correct diagnosis relatively little remains to be done for the patient. A combined diagnostic and therapeutic laparotomy is carried out at a time when secondary sexual characteristics of the female type are well developed, in order that the testes may be removed without producing an essential hormonal lack.

The choice of whether to remove the testes may be a difficult one, especially if the patient is not convinced of the necessity for doing so. After full maturation of the individual there is not much reason to preserve the feminizing testis, but the patient should be made aware that estrogen substitution will be a long-term necessity.

In some instances the surgical lengthening of the vagina improves the capability for sexual intercourse.

Most authors recommend that persons with feminizing testes be assigned the female sex.[8, 34] They already have near-normal feminine bodies, have in most cases been brought up as girls, and are functioning in female roles. In addition it is usually surgically next to impossible to transform these patients into males with any reasonable hope of successful function in society.

Gonadal Tumors

The patient with testicular feminization is likely to develop gonadal tumors because of the undescended status of the testis and its dysgenetic development. However, the seemingly high incidence of such tumors may be due in part to the fact that a patient with an unusual tumor is more likely to be the subject of medical investigation and a published case report. The types of neoplasms described below have been found.

Tubular adenomas are reported as being the most frequently occurring tumor. The distinction between nodular hyperplasia of the seminiferous tubules and true adenoma may at times be obscure. It is likely that opinions differ on the location of the boundary line between the two conditions. It is likely also that the gradually increasing amounts of proliferation make the hyperplastic nodule and the adenoma very closely related on the scale of growth activity. In general, the hyperplastic nodule is made up of normal units of the same size, orientation, and cellular composition. It is encapsulated to the extent that its enlarging causes compression of surrounding tissues. The nodules contain both immature seminiferous tubules and fetal-type Leydig cells. The adenoma is made up of units showing somewhat different elements, possibly more variable and less uniform in size and shape. It contains only tubules or tubules with an occasional Leydig cell. The adenoma is spheroidal with a fibrous tissue capsule, resembling an actual mass or tumor.

Leydig cell adenomas have been described in dysgenetic gonads and in testes. The distinction between nodular hyperplasia of Leydig cells and adenoma is difficult. The same generalities may be made regarding form, cellular make-up, and encapsulation in the case of interstitial proliferative lesions as in the case of tubular lesions.

Germinoma (dysgerminoma, seminoma) of the feminizing testis represents the most commonly encountered malignant tumor. Essentially the same tumor is found in both the ovary and the testis, but in the male it follows a more malignant clinical course. The germinoma is a tumor of the germ cell, in this case spermatogonium. Its presence in the dysgenetic testis is evidence that some of the elements in this type of organ are germ cells.

Embryonal carcinoma and teratoma have been found in the dysgenetic testis. Both are tumors of the germ cell series.[22, 33]

The reported high incidence of both benign and malignant tumors in testes of this type may be, again, somewhat biased. The interesting case history is more likely to appear in print. Accurate appraisal of the rate of occurrence awaits accumulation of more data.

Testicular feminization. BR-226028. (Patient of Drs. M. Schudmak and D. Gordon, Baton Rouge.) This 17-year-old Caucasian female was first seen by a surgeon because of a bulging mass in the left groin. She had just graduated from high school and planned to attend college in the fall. When the surgeon learned that she had not begun to menstruate, he referred her to a gynecologist. Examination showed the patient to be somewhat short in stature. Breast development was ample, although nipples and areolae were puerile. External genital organs were normally formed but immature. Clitoris and labia minora were small, like those of the prepubertal girl. Labia majora were smooth and rounded but displayed only a sparse hair growth. When the labia were held apart and the vaginal vestibule visualized, both vaginal and urethral orifices appeared normally formed and placed. The pink hymen was well-developed and was positioned at the vaginal opening. The vagina ended blindly at about 3 in. depth.

Hormonal assays on 24-hour urine specimen showed the following values: 17-ketosteroids, 22.2 mg; FSH, 50–100 MU; 17-ketogenic steroids, 9.9 mg; total estrogens, 17 g; and testosterone-epitestosterone, 855 g.

Thus it can be seen that the testosterone complex was extremely high, while the FSH was about the level found in castrates.

Sex chromatin was not seen in buccal cells, and the karyotype was 46 XY (Fig. 5-7).

A single surgical operation was carried out to repair the inguinal hernias (bilateral sacs were present) and to determine the type of gonads encountered. The internal genitalia consisted of two testes located at the internal inguinal rings, rudimentary or absent vas deferens and rudimentary or absent epididymis. No müllerian derivatives were seen. A transverse septum of peritoneum crossed the pelvic area from one gonad to the other. Wedge biopsy of the testes was done. The choice of whether to remove the intraabdominal testes was not

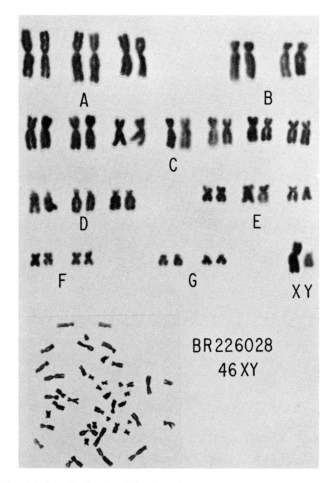

Fig. 5-7. Testicular feminization, karyotype 46 XY. BR-226028.

the surgeon's, as the patient requested that they not be taken out.

Microscopic examination of the testes showed nodular hyperplasia of the tubular element. Individual seminiferous tubules were of the fetal type without lumina and with immature Sertoli cells and few or no germ cells. Interstitial cells were gathered in aggregates about the periphery of nodules of tubules (Fig. 5-8).

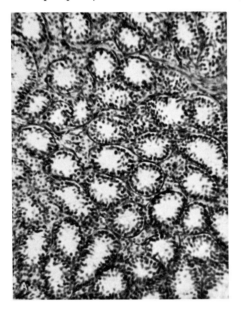

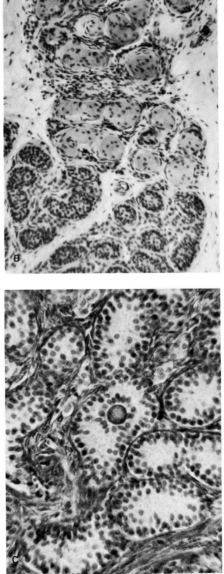

Fig. 5-8. Testicular feminization, BR-226028. *A*. Biopsy of intraabdominal testis showing immature seminiferous tubules with beginning lumen formation. There are relatively large numbers of interstitial cells. 70×. *B*. Focal area of hyalinization of seminiferous tubules. 70×. *C*. Seminiferous tubules lined by undifferentiated cells. One tubule contains calcium body. Interstitial cells are prominent. 480×.

Male Pseudohermaphroditism

Definition

Individuals with testes, usually ectopic in location, and incomplete masculinization, usually of the external genitalia, make up this group. They may come to the attention of the gynecologist because the external genitalia are more female than male in appearance, the breasts undergo female development at the time of puberty, and the incompletely masculinized male may possess uterus and fallopian tubes and may even "menstruate." [27]

The intersex individuals classed as male pseudohermaphrodites exhibit more variation than any other group. Indeed, it has been observed that as the general knowledge of intersex increases the number of patients classified as pseudohermaphrodites decreases.

Cause

A variety of factors may produce the condition. Probably a sex chromosomal abnormality with inadequate inductor causes poor embryonal and fetal testicular function.

Presenting Symptoms

Undescended testis, hernia, inadequate masculinization, sterility, or gynecomastia are the symptoms that prompt the patient to seek medical attention.

Testes

The gonads are testes though the degree of development and abnormalcy of these organs varies. Most often they are ectopically located, either in the inguinal canal or within the abdomen in the position where the ovaries would be found in a female. The testes are smaller than normal, but among published case reports no mention is made of absence of one testis. The diagnosis is suggested when routine examination indicates absence of scrotal testes.

Microscopic examination shows the testes to be dysgenetic. Tubules are immature, usually do not possess a lumen, and do not show evidence of germinal activity. Cells lining the seminiferous tubules are somewhat similar to the undifferentiated cells found in the feminizing testis. The majority of these cells are probably Sertoli cells, but spermatogonia have been noted.[27] Leydig cells are usually in evidence between tubules and in the hilar region. As expected, they are not as numerous in the pseudohermaphroditic testis as they are in the testis of testicular feminization, since Leydig cell hyperplasia is produced by gonadotropin stimulation.

Internal Genital Organs

Most male pseudohermaphrodites have internal genital ducts of müllerian origin, i.e., fallopian tubes and uterus; a few have no müllerian-derived structures; and some have both müllerian and wolffian derivatives. This seems to indicate that in its development the embryonic testis was unable to accomplish either of its two principal tasks: to inhibit the müllerian ducts or to stimulate sufficiently the wolffian ducts. It must, indeed, then, be classified as dysgenetic testis.

The tubes and uterus are of the infantile type. The uterus may be rudimentary, consisting of only muscular condensations without endometrial cavity. Sometimes the uterus does not connect to the rest of the genitourinary apparatus. Sometimes it connects by a short vagina to the "urethra"—actually the urogenital sinus—and thus has an opening to the outside.

When it is present the vas deferens may be palpated in the peritoneum of the broad ligament, its traditional location. It connects with the epididymis at the hilum of the testis and runs down beside the uterus, cervix, and vagina, ending in the region of the colliculus seminalis. In the lower, or caudal, region the vas may form an ampulla near the cervix or vagina, by which it opens into the urogenital sinus.

Urogenital Sinus and External Genitalia

In conditions in which the müllerian ductal structures persist, a vagina of sorts is usually formed. In the case of testicular feminization the vagina is, for all external appearances, normal. The hymen is in the proper relation with the urethral meatus, and both these openings communicate with the outside through the vaginal vestibule, the caudal remnant of the embryonic urogenital sinus. In male pseudohermaphroditism, however, the urogenital sinus (vaginal vestibule) is masculinized and converted into a tube by fusion of the urethral folds (labia minora). When the fusion is extensive, there is only a single opening to the outside. Urethral meatus and hymenal opening are not seen in their normal relation, but are both located somewhere at a depth within the urogenital sinus. In this condition the vagina is often said to open into the posterior (caudal) aspect of the urethra, a mistaken concept. Unless the vagina is very rudimentary, its connection with either the urogenital sinus or the vaginal vestibule is marked by the same structure—the hymen. Thus, the caudal end of the vagina can be easily identified.

The appearance of the external genitalia of the male pseudohermaphrodite varies greatly. Usually these structures are of almost normal male proportions. Hair distribution and phallus are of the normal masculine type. Usually the scrotal sacs are empty of testes on one or both sides;

when testes are present they are smaller than expected. The more masculinized individuals have a penile urethra, while those with more feminized genitalia have a single urogenital sinus opening at the base of the phallus.

Somatic Features

A frequently found abnormality is inguinal hernia, a feature reminiscent of the high incidence of hernia in some of the other forms of intersex. The relief of symptoms of hernia may be the patient's reason for seeking medical care. A small number of male pseudohermaphrodites have been found to have herniation of uterus and tubes within the inguinal hernia with or without vas deferens and testis on the same side.

Gynecomastia may appear when the male pseudohermaphrodite reaches puberty. Body and sexual hair are about the normal amount for males.

Hormonal Patterns

Since the group of male pseudohermaphrodites is a heterogeneous one, the hormonal patterns are also varied. In general the hormone levels are not distinctive. *Androgen* levels are normal in the prepubertal period and either slightly low or normal in the matured individual, the level correlating roughly with the masculinity or lack of it of the person himself. *Gonadotropin* levels are not greatly different from those of the normal male, except in the person with obviously inadequate testicular function, in whom they are higher than normal.

Chromosomal Patterns

The usual karyotype found in the male pseudohermaphrodite is 46 XY; thus if there is a chromosomal defect, it is not apparent at the present stage of our knowledge. Other individuals (e.g., patient CH56-236752) have the same pattern as the individual with mixed gonadal dysgenesis, i.e., 45 X0/46 XY. These two types of intersex are similar in other ways as well.

Differential Diagnosis

Male pseudohermaphroditism may be mistaken for true hermaphroditism, for mixed gonadal dysgenesis, or theoretically at least, for female pseudohermophroditism. Differentiation is based on karyotype: XY for male pseudohermaphroditism, XX for true hermaphroditism, mosaic pattern for mixed gonadal dysgenesis, and XX for female pseudohermaphroditism. In addition, the male pseudohermaphrodite has more masculine external genitalia, normal sexual hair, and bilateral testes.

Treatment

Treatment consists, after the diagnosis is ascertained, of adapting the individual to the appropriate sex. In the case of the male pseudohermaphrodite this consists usually of reinforcing the male characteristics and removing the female appurtenances. At laparotomy, the uterus and tubes are removed as superfluous. Externally the urinary conduit is made to follow its natural course whenever possible. If ectopic gonads are removed, hormonal substitution should be instituted as a long-term measure.

Gonadal Tumors

Since the testes in male pseudohermaphroditism are comparable to those in testicular feminization, they would be expected to develop the same types of tumors: tubular adenoma and adenomatous hyperplasia, germinoma, Leydig cell adenoma, and teratoma. The rates of occurrence of these tumors are not known, since their numbers are not large enough for calculation of rates.

Male pseudohermaphroditism. CH56-236752. A 3-month-old Caucasian was found on examination to have masculinized female external genitalia. Hypospadias and a vagina with a urethra opening into the anterior (ventral) wall were noted, but no mention was made of the position of the hymen. (This description is characteristic of persistent urogenital sinus.) The phallus was smaller than the normal male organ and was shaped with a caudal curvature. Redundant wrinkled skin simulated scrotum but no gonads were palpable within. There was a right inguinal hernia.

No sex chromatin was seen in cells of a buccal smear; 29 cell plates had 45 chromosomes while 7 plates had 46. Karyotype was 45 X0/46 XY (Figs. 5-9 and 5-10).

Combined herniorrhaphy and laparotomy were done. The hernia contained uterus, fallopian tubes, and two gonads. The surgeon thinking the gonads might be ovaries removed a small piece of each for biopsy. When both gonads were proved to be testes, a second surgical procedure was planned to bring down the testes. The surgeon succeeded only in removing the rudimentary uterus and tubes, describing the operation for undescended testes as hopeless because both would have to be brought down on the same side.

Both testicles showed immature or fetal-type seminiferous tubules, none of which contained lumina. There was focal calcification in a few tubules with slight thickening of the basement membrane. The

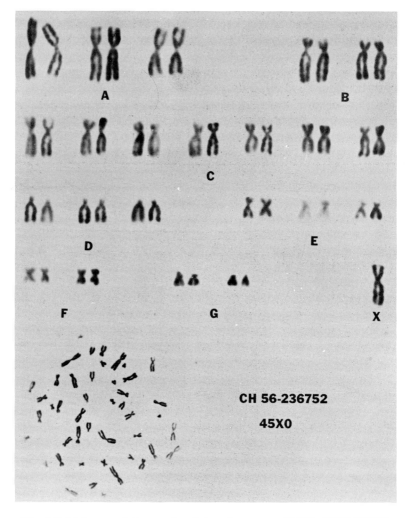

Fig. 5-9. Male pseudohermaphroditism, karyotype 45 X0. CH56-236752.

pattern of growth was suggestive of nodular hyperplasia, but no adenomas were seen. The few interstitial cells were not prominent. The tunica was well developed. The tubules were composed of undifferentiated cells and a few large clear cells suggestive of spermatogonia (Fig. 5-11).

Several surgical procedures were performed on the external genitalia to improve their function in a male role. The child was reared as a male.[7]

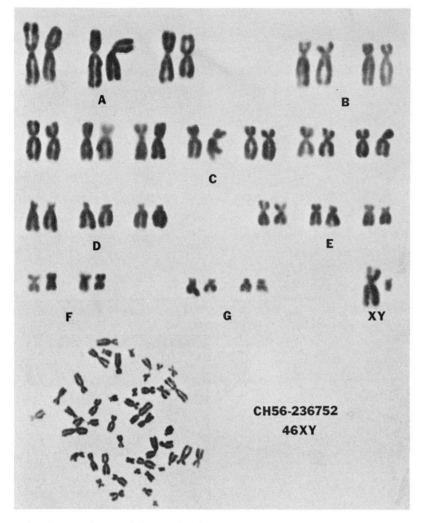

Fig. 5-10. Male pseudohermaphroditism, karyotype 46 XY. CH56-236752.

Klinefelter's Syndrome

As one of the defective testis syndromes this condition is of interest to the gynecologist because it continues the inadequate male spectrum begun with the syndrome of testicular feminization. In the short interval between discoveries of the nuclear sex chromatin mass and of the method for karyotyping human beings, the male with Klinefelter's syndrome was considered to be a gynecologic patient in that he had sex chromatin and was a genetic female.

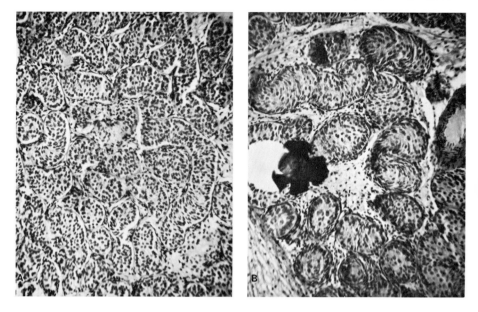

Fig. 5-11. Male pseudohermaphroditism. CH56-236752. *A*. Section of abdominal testis showing fetal type seminiferous tubules without lumina. Interstitial cells are present but decreased in number. 240×. *B*. Dysgenetic gonad with small calcium body in seminiferous tubule. 240×.

Definition

As reported by its discoverer, Klinefelter's syndrome is "characterized by gynecomastia, aspermatogenesis without a-Leydigism, and increased excretion of follicle-stimulating hormone."[18]

Cause

The condition results from a sex chromosomal abnormality (polyploidy-X) causing primary tubular and germ cell atrophy.

Presenting Symptom

The disorder may be discovered incidentally or suspected on the basis of gynecomastia or infertility.

Gonads

The testes are the site of the primary abnormality. They are always located in the scrotum, a feature setting Klinefelter's syndrome apart from male pseudohermaphroditism, in which the testes are often ectopically located. Each testis measures about 1.5 by 1 cm and is of normal consistency and sensitivity. A normal amount of semen is produced by the accessory glands, but it is made up of fluid without sperm.

Microscopic examination of testicular tissue or biopsy specimens reveals the lesion to be primary testicular atrophy. Seminiferous tubules are sclerotic, and sheaths of the tubules are thickened and hyalinized. In focal areas the fibrosis and sclerosis are not complete, seemingly allowing viability and the opportunity for functioning on the part of the tubular epithelium. In these areas the tubular epithelium appears to be made up mostly of Sertoli cells. Some of the tubules possess lumina, a few have identifiable germinal elements, and in rare instances there is spermatogenesis.[32] Leydig cells appear to undergo hyperplastic proliferation, although it is difficult to assess whether there is an actual increase in the number compared with the normal organ or only a proportionate increase due to the small size of the testis. There are three recognizable indicators of activity of the Leydig cells: (1) cytoplasmic inclusions of Reinke may be seen, (2) electron microscopic indicators of cellular activity are present, and (3) lipoid material in the cytoplasm can be demonstrated by histochemical staining. There is definite morphologic evidence of loss of functional activity after suppression of pituitary gonadotropin.[3, 30]

Internal Genital Organs

Vas deferens and prostate are similar to those of the normal male. No müllerian structures have been reported in those individuals whose internal genital organs have been inspected.

External Genitalia

The prepubertal child with Klinefelter's syndrome has apparently normal genitalia. The penis is of average size and the testes are not significantly smaller than normal. With the onset of maturation, the small size of the testes become evident. Pubic and sexual hair are male type. The penis is of a small normal proportion and erections are possible.

Somatic Features

Gynecomastia is found in most but not all persons with Klinefelter's syndrome. Though not pendulus, the breasts are beyond question of a feminine contour. The major part of the enlargement is said to take place in the connective tissue rather than in the parenchymal tissues of the breasts.[17, 18] No other stigmata are associated with the genital lesions of Klinefelter's syndrome. There are, however, signs of underdevelopment of secondary sex characteristics as a result of testicular inadequacy and of changes such as osteoporosis due to insufficient production of androgenic hormone.

Hormonal Patterns

In practically all patients with Klinefelter's syndrome pituitary FSH levels are increased to the level found in the castrate state. This finding is so constant that Klinefelter himself considered it a diagnostic *sine qua non*. The high FSH may easily be suppressed with testosterone or oral estrogen. The urinary excretion of *androgens* is normal or definitely below normal. Estrogen levels are usually low; in an occasional patient they are those of a normal woman.

Chromosomal Patterns

In males with Klinefelter's syndrome there is a sex chromatin mass in nuclei of cells scraped from the buccal cavity. This finding initially gave the false impression that these patients were females, whereas it may be recalled that the chromatin mass is actually a polyploid X chromosome.

The minimal chromosomal complement in Klinefelter's syndrome is 47 XXY. Individuals with the Klinefelter somatotype but with a karyotype of 46 XY are considered to have "false" Klinefelter's syndrome. Individuals with karyotypes of XXY and one or two extra X chromosomes, and males with XXY plus an extra Y or X and Y, have the phenotype of Klinefelter's syndrome but an aggregate number of chromosomes of 47, 48, or 49. In general, the higher the chromosomal number the greater the degree of mental retardation.

Treatment

In individuals with signs of hypogonadism it is important to administer androgen therapy. The patient should understand that this measure is on a permanent basis. The gynecomastia may be treated by surgical excision of the breast if desirable.

Gonadal Tumors

There is no reported predisposition to develop tumors of the testes. However, since the testes of the person with Klinefelter's syndrome are dysgenetic and show nodular hyperplasia of the interstitial cells, a higher rate of tumorigenesis is possible and periodic examination is prudent.

Klinefelter's syndrome (testicular tubular atrophy). CH54-136262. (Patient of Dr. W. G. Blackard, Louisiana State University School of

Medicine, New Orleans.) On examination, a 16-year-old Negro was found to have small and soft testes, the left one being "poorly formed." A small amount of breast tissue was palpable in the enlarged breasts bilaterally. Although the patient was of a muscular build, the proportions of body and extremities appeared eunuchoid.

There was no difficulty in identifying genitals and somatic features as male type. Pubic and axillary hair were present. The phallus was an essentially normal male organ. Apparently, the patient was capable of erection but was reluctant to discuss sexual activities. Both testes were normally placed within the scrotum.

Cells in the buccal smear contained a single sex chromatin mass. Karyotype prepared from lymphocyte culture showed a chromosomal complement of 47 XXY (Fig. 5-12).

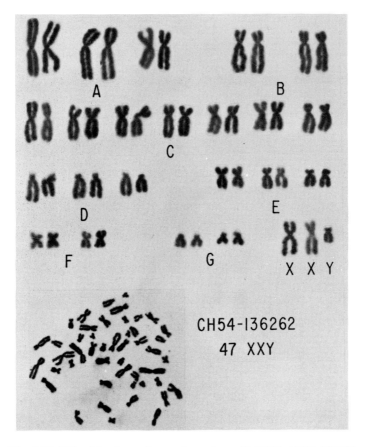

Fig. 5-12. Klinefelter's syndrome, karyotype 47 XXY. CH54-136262.

The patient's mental status was estimated to be slightly below average, but possibly this impression was due to his retiring personality. The patient declined testicular biopsy.

Ovary-Testis Syndrome: True Hermaphroditism

Definition

A single individual having both ovary and testis is a true hermaphrodite. The arrangement of gonadal elements has been reported in all possible combinations, including ovary and testis on the same or opposite sides and one or two ovotestes with both elements in the same organ.

Cause

The cause is unknown. Chromosomal malfunction or failure in the process of gonadal corticomedullary differentiation may be responsible. Several different factors may be involved. In persons having ovotestis, the condition may represent an atavism, as gonads of that kind are found in some lower species.

Presenting Symptoms

Inadequate masculinization at puberty, breast development in an apparent male at puberty, menstruation in an apparent male, or amenorrhea in an apparent female at puberty may prompt medical consultation.

Gonads

The gonads may be found in any location from the intraabdominal site to the scrotal site. In general, if the gonad is testis it is likely to be scrotal or inguinal or associated with an inguinal hernia. If the gonad is ovary it is likely to be in the customary location or in the cul-de-sac. If ovarian tissue is found in the scrotum, the gonad is probably ovotestis, since the ovary is seldom located outside of the abdomen. Testes are usually identified by their smooth white tunica and epididymis, while ovary is fairly distinctive in appearance. The ovotestis cannot, however, be reliably identified by its visual characteristics and may be mistaken for either testis or ovary.

The microscopic structures of the separate testis and ovary are not greatly different from those of the normal organs. The scrotal testis may be like the normal testis, even to the point of producing spermatozoa, a feature which authenticates the type of the gonad without necessity for biopsy. The intraabdominal testis is apt to be somewhat dysgenetic in that the tubules are immature, are made up of undifferentiated cells or Sertoli cells, and are fibrotic in large areas. There are no lumina in the tubules.

The basement membrane of the tubules is thickened. In better developed testes spermatogonia can be identified. Reports indicate that the interstitial cells are absent, normal, or increased in number. Presumably, the presence or absence of Leydig cells correlates with the masculinity or lack of it in the particular individual. When the testes are more differentiated and matured, there usually are mesonephric derivatives at the hilum.

The separate ovary, like the separate testis, is less than perfect. Follicular and germinal elements are necessarily present, their development or lack of development roughly paralleling the norm for chronologic age of the individual at the time of examination. The histologic diagnosis of ovary cannot reliably be made upon the finding of ovarian cortical stromal tissue without follicles and ova. In the ovarian hilum prominent rete ovarii and mesonephric remnants are often noted. Corpora lutea may be present in the ovary of the hermaphrodite who menstruates.[2, 27]

The ovotestis, that curious combination gonad found in humans only in the intersex individual but in many lesser animals as standard equipment, is usually polarized, with ovarian structures at one pole and testicular parts at the other. The dividing line is not always sharp, however, and tubules may be found within ovarian cortex and primordial follicles within the testicular fibrous tissue. The respective gonadal tissues in the ovotestis are more dysgenetic than those of the separate gonads. The tubules of the testicular portion are of the immature type without lumina, while the cellular component is made up of undifferentiated cells or Sertoli cells without germinal elements. The ovarian portion is more fibrotic with fewer primordial follicles evident. The dominance of the ovarian or the testicular portion of the ovotestis is consonant, usually, with the corresponding chromosomal complement, i.e., the XY individual shows better testicular differentiation, while the XX person has better ovarian differentiation.

Gonadal Tumors

Although the gonads of the true hermaphrodite for the most part are severely dysgenetic, case reports do not indicate a high incidence of gonadal tumors. Of the several types found, the germinoma is the usual one, and may be noted in ovotestes or testes.

Among ovarian enlargements most frequently found are the non-neoplastic cystic follicular tumors.

Because the gonads are abnormal and because many of these individuals have ectopic testes or testicular tissue, the examiner should be alert to the possibility of tumor formation, in spite of the apparently low rate of occurrence.

Internal Genital Organs

Uterus and one or two fallopian tubes are present in most true hermaphrodites. Often the uterus is incompletely formed, bicornuate or unicornuate, reflecting the partial or unilateral operation of the müllerian-
inhibiting action of the hermaphroditic fetal testis. Jones pointed out
that the uterine abnormalities are greater in the case of patients with
bilateral ovotestes.[13]

Fallopian tube develops on the side with an ovary, and also develops
more often than vas deferens when the gonad is ovotestis. Vas deferens
and epididymis are induced on the side of the testis. Occasionally, both
vas deferens and fallopian tube are formed on the same side or bilaterally; both may be rudimentary. Palpation of the prostate gland indicates
a rudimentary or small organ or occasionally a gland of approximately
normal size.

External Genitalia

These structures are usually female or female-like, with enlargement
of the phallus, but in some patients the organs are nearly normally male.
All intermediate forms between these two extremes have been seen.
The phallus may appear to be an undersized penis without a penile
urethra. The opening at the base of the phallus transmits urine and in
some instances menstrual fluid. Masculinized female genitalia also show
partial labial fusion with wrinkling and redundancy of the skin of the
labia majora, simulating scrotum. Pubic hair is normal. Vaginal vestibule and vagina are compromised to varying degrees with other effects of
masculinization. Although usually of about normal proportions the vagina may be infantile or rudimentary. Some reports state that the vagina
"opens into the urethra" or the urethra "opens into the vagina"; these
are false concepts indicating that both open into a persistent urogenital
sinus. The scrotum may contain one or no gonads, only very exceptionally
both organs. There is frequently an inguinal hernia, and this sac may
contain a cryptorchid testis or ovotestis.

Common conditions found in males which must be differentiated from
the changes due to hermaphroditism are hypospadias, cryptorchidism,
and cleft scrotum.

Somatic Features

The true hermaphrodite is of normal stature and build, and except
for external genital organs no stigma of intersex is reflected in the
somatotype before puberty. A majority of individuals develop enlargement of the breasts at sexual maturity and nearly half undergo cyclic

uterine bleeding, which may be misinterpreted in the "male" as hematuria. Probably because most true hermaphrodites have enlargement of the phallus, the majority are reared as males; this choice is reinforced later by the fact that most develop male-like musculature and male sexual hair.

Hormone Pattern

No specific changes from the normal hormonal pattern are observed in true hermaphrodites. Both *estrogen* and *androgen* excretion may be within the normal range or slightly low, the amounts of these hormones being roughly proportional to the amount of ovarian or testicular tissue and its differentiation and to the predominant somatotype. *Pituitary FSH* is normal in the young person, probably indicating gonadal function in steroid hormone production.

Ovulation has been noted, and the finding of a corpus luteum in either ovary or ovotestis proves this event. However, fertility has not been proved by conception and pregnancy. Similarly, although spermatogenesis may rarely be found, fatherhood has not been proved.

Chromosomal Patterns

It has been estimated from published reports that two-thirds of true hermaphrodites have the normal female chromosomal complement, 46 XX. Most of the remainder have the 46 XY pattern. The most interesting mosaic pattern noted is 46 XX/XY. Governed by the chromosomal make-up, sex chromatin is present (female type) in most individuals, absent (male type) in most of the rest, and present with reduced count (chromosomal mosaicism) in a few.

In general, there is a rough correlation among the chromosomal complement, the predominant gonadal tissue, the external genitalia, and the hormone pattern. The correlation does not extend to the sex of rearing, however, for although most true hermaphrodites have the 46 XX pattern, most are reared as males.

Behavioral Patterns

Since most true hermaphrodites are assigned the male sex and reared as males, there is a proportionate number whose major gonadal component and chromosomal component do not agree with the sex of rearing. It has been observed that most of these persons are satisfied with their assignment. If the treatment of the hermaphrodite contemplates a reversal of sex to accord more closely with gonadal and secondary sexual characteristics, the change must be made very early in life, possibly by the age of 2 years. At older ages the patient does not make completely satisfactory psychologic adjustment to sex reversal.

Treatment

When true hermaphroditism is diagnosed at the time of adolescence or maturity, it is psychologically important to preserve the assigned sex of the individual and to carry out surgical procedures which reinforce that sex. It should be kept in mind, however, in that the hermaphrodite may elect not to try to adapt to either male or female role in a family setting, but quietly to keep the in-between status and lead a platonic, solo, or nonfamily life.

Surgical procedures of value are those for removing unnecessary contradictory sex organs, such as uterus and tubes in the apparent male. Surgical removal of the abdominal testis or the ovotestis is advisable, since the dysgenetic gonad may be the site of tumor formation. Plastic repair and reconstruction of the external genitalia must be done early, soon after diagnosis has been established and a total plan of management outlined. These procedures are the more urgent if the relation of vagina, urethra, and urogenital sinus are such that there is improper function in urination or retention of urine in bladder or vagina.

Timing of the surgical removal of the gonads is important. Too early removal allows eunuchoid development of the skeleton and prevents development of secondary sex characteristics, including mature moods and attitudes. The prospect of breast development may be highly desirable or equally highly detestable, depending upon the chosen sex of rearing of the individual.

Hormonal substitution therapy has a definite place in treatment. In the female estrogen substitution assures continued maintenance of the female habitus, while in the male testosterone administration promotes masculinization.

True hermaphroditism. CH54-153672. This year-old Negro infant was examined when the parents could not decide whether it was a boy or a girl. The external genitalia consisted of a short phallus curved caudally, a "urethra" opening at the base of the phallus, and a scrotum containing a right testis. There was no gonad in the left scrotum. When examined under anesthesia the patient was found to have a small vagina.

Sex chromatin was present in somatic cells. Chromosomal complement was 46 XX (Fig. 5-13). 17-Ketosteroids were 2.5 and 1.1 mg/24 hours (low normal). Intravenous pyelography was normal.

Laparotomy was done to determine presence and type of internal

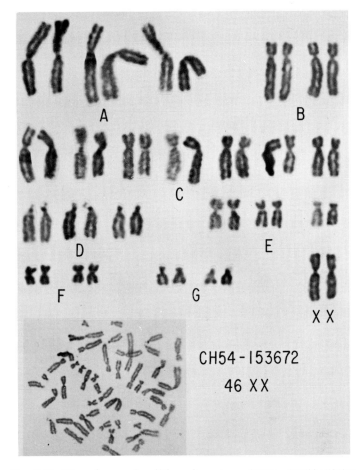

Fig. 5-13. True hermaphroditism, karyotype 46XX. CH54-153672.

genital organs, especially left gonad. The surgeon described a left ovary and tube but did not positively identify a uterus. Since the child was being reared as a boy and since the external genitalia looked more male than female, the surgeon elected to remove the ovary and tube. The testicle was biopsied.

Histologic study of the specimens showed ovary with many primordial follicles, testicle with immature seminiferous tubules containing no spermatogonia and few Leydig cells, and an enlarged area of the fallopian tube which resembled an infantile uterus (Fig. 5-14).

Much later, the patient underwent corrective procedures to reinforce male function.

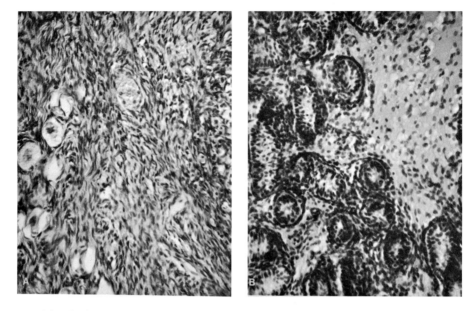

Fig. 5-14. True hermaphroditism. CH54-153672. *A.* Ovary and primordial follicles located on left side in normal location of ovary. 240×. *B.* Biopsy of right scrotal gonad showing immature seminiferous tubules. 240×.

SURGICAL OPERATIONS UPON THE EXTERNAL GENITALIA

General considerations in the choice of surgical operation upon the female external genitalia are similar in the several types of intersex inasmuch as the deformities of the genitals are similar. Descriptive terminology common to the basic types of intersex include: (1) *contradictory genitalia,* in which the gonadal or chromosomal sex is of one type while the external genitalia are of the opposite type; (2) *masculinized female genitalia,* in which there are various degrees of clitoral hypertrophy, deepening of the fossa navicularis by fusion of the labia minora, and redundancy and wrinkling of the skin of the labia majora; and (3) inadequate or *incompletely masculinized male genitalia,* in which there are somewhat undersized penis, chordee, absence of penile urethra, and perhaps cryptorchidism.

Purpose of Operation

Since only a few hermaphrodites possess the actual or potential ability to reproduce, surgical operation is aimed at improving capability for coitus. Occasionally improvement of the appearance of the external genitalia is the chief consideration. In a few cases, urinary drainage must be improved to prevent back pressure and stasis in the lower urinary tract.

Timing

Selection of the proper time in the development and growth of the person is of prime importance. Corrections must be made before the individual is old enough to have appreciable insight into his deformity, but plastic operations upon small parts may present insurmountable technical difficulties. Certain procedures may be successful in the presence of favorable hormonal balance of the older intersex person. Reconstruction of the vagina, for example, should be delayed until the age of sexual maturity.

Psychologic Factors

Surgical changes aimed at altering or reversing the somatic sex require detailed explanation and intensive consideration by physician and parents as well as by the patient himself. Experience has shown that the individual probably does not make satisfactory adjustment to sex reversal after the ages of 3 to 5 years. The importance of parental adjustment or lack of adjustment in such a situation should not be underestimated.

Types of Operations

The easiest surgical procedure and a valuable one is *biopsy of the gonads*. If the time is not right for removal of gonads, but a sound diagnosis is not obtainable without knowledge of gonadal histology, wedge biopsy or needle biopsy may supply the correct answers. If the surgeon chooses to remove one gonad while leaving the other he should take a sample of the organ to be left in place. Failure to perform this simple step may result in lack of information necessitating another major surgical procedure.

The operation most frequently used (both correctly and incorrectly) is *removal of the gonad*. The surgeon must keep in mind that this is an irreversible procedure. Further, he should know that even the dysgenetic gonad may contribute to the early growth and development of the individual. The choice of when to remove or whether to remove the gonad must be decided on the basis of what is best for the patient.

High on the list of corrective surgical procedures is *amputation of the hypertrophied clitoris*. Before he recommends amputation, the surgeon should ascertain that the organ is, indeed, grossly and unacceptably enlarged in the patient who is going to be reared as a female. In the case of lesser enlargement he would be better advised to wait. Removal of part of the clitoris should be done in a manner that preserves a part of the skin of the undersurface of the shaft with its nerve endings to form a small eminence. The shaft is exposed as far as the division of the crura, where both corpora are transsected.

Surgical correction is mandatory when the vagina and urethra join in a common urogenital sinus leading to the exterior. Elimination of the urogenital sinus and *creation of a vaginal vestibule* are not always easily done. The success of the operation is related to the severity of the deformity, i.e., the depth of the common urogenital sinus. When the caudal extent of the vagina, i.e., the point of formation of the hymen, can be brought down and joined to the exterior surface, the repair operation is likely to be successful. When the opening of the vagina is too far inside the urogenital sinus to reach the exterior surface, operation is usually unsuccessful. Careful preoperative study is necessary for appraisal of these possibilities.

Surgical improvement of the phallus can be done to make it look and function like a penis. *Release of chordee and construction of penile urethra* both help to some extent. It must be stated, however, that these and other procedures designed to strengthen a male predominance have certain in-built limitations.

REFERENCES

1. BARNES, A. C. *Intra-Uterine Development.* Philadelphia, Lea & Febiger, 1968, p. 264.
2. BREWER, J. I., JONES, H. D. J., and CULVER, H. True hermaphroditism. *JAMA 148:*431, 1952.
3. BURT, A. S., REINER, L., COHEN, R. B., and SNIFFEN, R. C. Klinefelter's syndrome: Report of autopsy with particular reference to histochemistry of the endocrine glands. *J Clin Endocrinol Metab 14:*719, 1954.
4. CAMPBELL, M. F., and HARRISON, J. H. (eds.). *Urology,* vol. 2. Philadelphia, Saunders, 1970, p. 1625.
5. CARR, D. H., HAGGAR, R. A., and HART, A. G. Germ cells in the ovaries of X0 female infants. *Am J Clin Pathol 49:*521, 1968.
6. COUNSELLER, V. S., NICHOLS, D. R., and SMITH, H. L. Congenital absence of testis. *J Urol 44:*237, 1940.
7. DOUGHERTY, C. M. *Surgical Pathology of Gynecologic Disease.* New York, Harper & Row, 1968, pp. 658–659.
8. FEDERMAN, D. D. *Abnormal Sexual Development: A Genetic and Endocrine Approach to Differential Diagnosis.* Philadelphia, Saunders, 1967, pp. 50, 55, 68, 72, 89, 110, 183.
9. FORD, C. E. The Cytogenetics of Human Intersexuality. In Overzier, C. (ed.). *Intersexuality.* New York, Academic Press, 1963, p. 113.
10. HAUSER, G. A. Testicular Feminization. In Overzier, C., *op. cit.,* pp. 258, 267, 269, 300.

11. JONES, H. W. In discussion of Morris, J. M., and Mahesh, V. B. Further observations on the syndrome, "testicular feminization." *Am J Obstet Gynecol 87*:747, 1963.

12. JONES, H. W., FERGUSON-SMITH, M. A., and HELLER, R. H. The pathology and cytogenetics of gonadal agenesis. *Am J Obstet Gynecol 87*:578, 1963.

13. JONES, H. W., JR., and SCOTT, W. W. *Hermaphroditism, Genital Anomalies and Related Endocrine Disorders.* Baltimore, Williams & Wilkins, 1958, p. 93.

14. JONES, H. W., JR., and VERKAUF, B. S. Surgical treatment in congenital adrenal hyperplasia. *Obstet Gynecol 36*:1, 1970.

15. JOST, A., and BOZIC, B. Données sur la differentiation des conduits genitaux du foetus de rat etudiée in vitro. *CR Soc Biol (Paris) 145*:647, 1951.

16. JOST, A. Embryonic Sexual Differentiation (Morphology, Physiology, Abnormalities). In Jones, H. W., Jr., and Scott, W. W., *op. cit.,* p. 24.

17. KLINEFELTER, H. F., JR. Klinefelter's Syndrome. In Jones, H. W., Jr., and Scott, W. W., *op. cit.,* p. 85.

18. KLINEFELTER, H. F., JR., REIFENSTEIN, E. C., JR., and ALBRIGHT, F. A syndrome characterized by gynecomastia, aspermatogenesis without a-Leydigism and increased excretion of follicle stimulating hormone. *J Clin Endocrinol Metab 2*:615, 1942.

19. LEESON, C. R., SMITH, B. D., and BUNGE, R. G. Microscopic appearance of the gonads in prepubertal male intersex individuals simulating females. *Invest Urol 5*:361, 1968.

20. LYON, M. F. Sex chromatin and gene action in the mammalian X-chromosome. *Am J Hum Genet 14*:135, 1962.

21. McKUSICK, V. On the X chromosome in man. *Q Rev Biol 37*:69, 1962.

22. MELICOW, M. M. Tumors of dysgenetic gonads in intersexes. *Bull NY Acad Med 42*:3, 1966.

23. MORRIS, J. M. The syndrome of testicular feminization in male pseudohermaphrodites. *Am J Obstet Gynecol 65*:1192, 1953.

24. MORRIS, J. M., and MAHESH, V. B. Further observations on the syndrome "testicular feminization." *Am J Obstet Gynecol 87*:731, 1963.

25. MORRIS, J. M., and SCULLY, R. E. *Endocrine Pathology of the Ovary.* St. Louis, Mosby, 1958.

26. O'LEARY, J. A. Comparative studies of the gonad in testicular feminization and cryptorchidism. *Fertil Steril 16*:813, 1965.

27. OVERZIER, C. (ed.). *Intersexuality.* New York, Academic Press, 1963, p. 208.

28. SCULLY, R. E. Gonadoblastoma: A gonadal tumor related to the dysgerminoma (seminoma) and capable of sex hormone production. *Cancer 6*:455, 1953.

29. SINGH, R. P., and CARR, D. H. The anatomy and histology of X0 human embryos and fetuses. *Anat Rec 155*:369, 1966.

30. SMITH, B. D., LEESON, C. R., and BUNGE, R. G. Microscopic appearance of the testis in Klinefelter's syndrome before and after suppression of gonadotrophin production with testosterone. *Invest Urol 5*:58, 1967.

31. SOHVAL, A., and SOFFER, L. Congenital familial testicular deficiency. *Am J Med 14*:328, 1953.

32. STEINBERGER, E., SMITH, K. D., and PERLOFF, W. H. Spermatogenesis in Klinefelter's Syndrome. *J Clin Endocrinol Metab 25*:1325, 1965.

33. TAYLOR, H., BARTER, R., and JACOBSON, C. B. Neoplasms of dysgenetic gonads. *Am J Obstet Gynecol 96*:816, 1966.
34. TETER, J., BULSKA, M., and RUSZKOWSKI, J. Pseudohermaphroditisme masculin avec feminisation particulierement marqué. *Bull Soc R Belge Gynecol Obstet 31*:1, 1961.
35. TETER, J., and TARLOWSKI, R. Tumors of the gonads in cases of gonadal dysgenesis and male pseudohermaphroditism. *Am J Obstet Gynecol 79*:321, 1960.
36. TURNER, H. H. A syndrome of infantilism, congenital webbed neck and cubitus valgus. *Endocrinology 23*:566, 1938.
37. WITSCHI, E. Embryogenesis of the adrenal and the reproductive glands. *Recent Progr Horm Res 6*:1, 1951.
38. WITSCHI, E. Fundamental Aspects of Intersexuality. In Overzier, C. (ed.), *op. cit.*, p. 18.
39. WITSCHI, E., and MENGERT, W. F. Endocrine studies on human hermaphrodites and their bearing on the interpretation of homosexuality. *J Clin Endocrinol Metab 2*:279, 1942.

Chapter Six

Unusual
Ovarian Development

John C. Weed

ABNORMAL CHROMOSOMAL PATTERNS

Various degrees of maldevelopment of the ovary occur in those phenotypic females with abnormal sex chromosomal patterns other than the well-known 45 X0 karyotype and 45 X0/46 XX mosaicism. These individuals may have one normal X chromosome plus an abnormal second X chromosome. The abnormality may be deletion of the long or the short arm, a small X, or an isochromosome of X; the last is the most common.[6]

Such patients consult a physician because of amenorrhea, delayed puberty with inadequate development of sexual characteristics, or a transient menstrual pattern after menarche. In general, those who have periodic bleeding manifest no abnormality in growth pattern and do not differ from the averages for height and weight in the normal female growth curves. Secondary sex characteristics are absent or poorly developed; breasts are small or rudimentary, genital and axillary hair is sparse, and both internal and external genitalia are infantile. In some instances epiphyseal fusion has been delayed in the long bones and pelvic bones many years beyond the expected age of closure.

Primary ovarian failure, karyotype 46 XXp—. OCHS 124-869. A 24-year-old white woman began menstruating between the ages of 12 and 13 and had six menstrual cycles at about 30-day intervals, lasting 5 to 6 days. She had reached her present growth at the age of 14 years. She had been slender prepubertally, then had become overweight, reaching a maximum weight of 173 lb.

Physical examination showed her height to be 59¼ in., her span 56¼ in., and her weight 159 lb. Her breasts were described as "small and normal." Her abdomen was obese. Axillary and pubic hair were normal in distribution. The hymen was intact; external genitalia were infantile. One examiner noted her appearance to be that characteristic of Turner's syndrome. Both fifth metacarpal bones were short.

X-ray studies of the sella turcica were normal. Incomplete fusion of the ossification centers of the iliac bones was seen on excretory urography, which was otherwise normal. Buccal smear revealed no sex chromatin. Her hemoglobin level was 13 g; hematocrit was 40 per cent. 17-Hydroxysteroid excretion was 6.6 mg/24 hours. Pituitary FSH was 50–100 mu/24 hours. Protein-bound iodine was 16.8 g/100 ml and the glucose tolerance test revealed a diabetic curve. Urinary excretion studies revealed testosterone 4.22 g/24 hours and epitestosterone 2.99 g/24 hours—both low values for this laboratory. Chromosome study revealed an abnormal female karyotype with consistent deletion of the short arms of one of the sex chromosomes (Fig. 6-1).

Laparotomy was refused. Replacement with estrogenic hormone has led to regular withdrawal bleeding and an improvement of emotional problems. Diabetes has been controlled with diet.

Primary ovarian failure, karyotype 46 Xx. OCHS 150-184. This white female patient was seen at the age of 16 years 10 months because of failure to grow, amenorrhea, and absence of secondary sexual development. She had been a normal, full-term infant, weighing 7 lb at birth, but was said to have been small all her life. She had done well in school.

Her height was 56¼ in. and her weight 80 lb. She had no breast development, no axillary or pubic hair, and infantile genitalia. She had an exaggerated carrying angle in her arm and a shield chest.

A 24-hour urine collection revealed gonadotropic hormones in excess of 96 MU/24 hours. Her hemoglobin was 12.5 g. Blood chemistries were within normal limits. 17-Ketosteroid level was 5.1 mg/24 hours.

Exploratory laparotomy revealed normal kidney development and rudimentary fallopian tubes and uterus. On the right, there was a streak ovary, but no ovarian tissue could be found on the left side. The ovarian streak was not removed.

Cyclic administration of conjugated estrogens was begun, and the patient continued to grow over a 10-year period to 59½ in. During

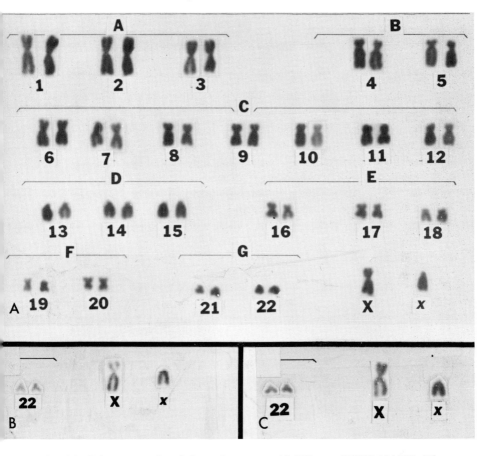

Fig. 6-1. Primary ovarian failure, karyotype 46 XXp−. OCHS 124-869. The abnormality consists of loss of short arms of one of the X chromosomes, a change found consistently in all three karyotypes.

this time her breasts developed and she grew normal pubic and axillary hair. Normal menstrual cycles developed, requiring supplementation with a progestogen, and subsequently a change to combination estrogen-progestogen tablets which regulated her menses.

Twelve years after initial examination, buccal and vaginal smears showed no sex chromatin. Karyotype was 46 Xx (Fig. 6-2).

In each of these cases the sex chromatin (Barr body) was absent. According to some reports [6] the sex chromatin reflects the chromatin mass in the second X chromosome—it is absent in X0 and minimal in Xxp− and Xx patterns.

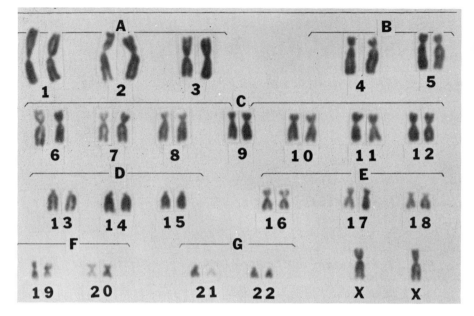

Fig. 6-2. Primary ovarian failure, karotype 46Xx. OCHS 150-184.

The similarity of the second case to Turner's (45 X0) syndrome is marked, and the anatomic findings are comparable. The small x chromosome and the X with deleted short arms therefore seem to be deficient in the genes which complete ovarian maturation and development.

Jacobs et al.,[2] who had a similar patient, have suggested that the genes which influence height are present on the short arms of the X chromosome, which are absent or diminished in these cases.

Primary amenorrhea may have other causes than those associated with chromosome abnormalities; however, the reports of Jacobs et al.[2] and Kadotani et al.[3] indicate that 38–43 per cent of phenotypic females with primary amenorrhea also have chromosomal abnormalities. For this reason, a chromosome study is indicated with this diagnosis.

NORMAL FEMALE CHROMOSOMAL PATTERNS

A second group of patients have inadequate ovarian development, normal female chromosomal patterns, and primary amenorrhea.

Primary amenorrhea, karyotype 46 XX in sisters. OCHS 273-319. A 19-year-old white female patient had apparently normal growth and development but her breasts did not develop. Pubic and axillary hair appeared at about 14 years of age. She had no acne. She was one of six siblings. One sister was normally developed at age 15 but still amenorrheic; the other sister at age 18 was amenorrheic.

The patient's height was 68¾ in., her span 71½ in., and her weight 103 lb. There was no breast development. The axillary hair was scanty. The vulva was infantile with scanty pubic hair. The vagina was of normal depth, but the mucosa was hypoestrogenic.

X-ray examination of the sella turcica was reported as normal. The capitofemoral epiphyses and those of the greater trochanter of the femurs were still present, revealing delayed maturation. Buccal smear showed sex chromatin. Intravenous pyelography was normal. Protein-bound iodine was 4.8 g/100 ml. FSH was more than 192 and less than 288 MU/24 hours. 17-Ketosteroid level was 9.3 mg/24 hours. Glucose tolerance test was within normal limits. Chromosome study revealed a normal diploid female karyotype, 46 XX (Fig. 6-3).

On culdoscopy an infantile uterus with normal tubes was found. Both ovaries were small, approximately 1 by 1.5 cm, and grossly inactive.

Her 18-year-old sister, with primary amenorrhea, studied 2 years later, also had a 46 XX karyotype with elevated FSH level. Physical development of the two sisters was similar, except that the younger

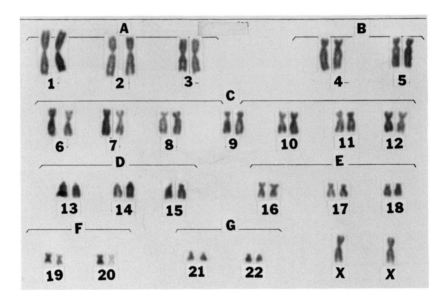

Fig. 6-3. Primary amenorrhea, karyotype 46 XX. OCHS 273-319.

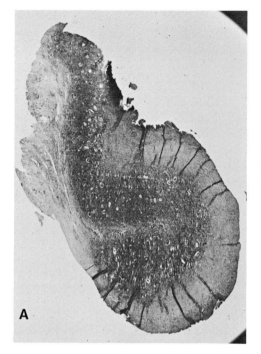

Fig. 6-4. Ovarian maldevelopment. OCHS 391-164. *A.* Cross-section of hypoplastic ovary measured 5 mm. Very few ova are seen. 10×. *B.* Primordial follicles spaced widely apart in ovarian cortex. 240×.

was shorter (61½ in.) and had delayed epiphyseal closure of her long bones.

Primary amenorrhea, karyotype 46 XX in sisters. OCHS 391-164. This white female patient, 23 years of age, had primary amenorrhea. Her first menstrual period was induced at the age of 17 by hormone administration, and all succeeding periods required preliminary hormonal therapy. She had no bleeding on progesterone administration nor did she respond to clomiphene. The FSH level, determined elsewhere, was said to have exceeded 50 MU/24 hours. Breast development followed the administration of hormones, but was absent at initial examination. She has had satisfactory menses following administration of ovarian replacement hormones (birth control pills).

Physical examination showed her height to be 61 in. and her weight 120½ lb. Her breasts were underdeveloped. There was little axillary hair. The vulva was normal without clitoral hypertrophy. The vaginal mucosa was hypoestrogenic; the cervix small and patent; and the uterus small. No adnexa could be outlined.

The laboratory examination was essentially normal. Sex chromatin was present. 17-Ketosteroid level was 8.8 mg/24 hours and FSH level was 100 MU/24 hours. Her karyotype was normal female, 46 XX.

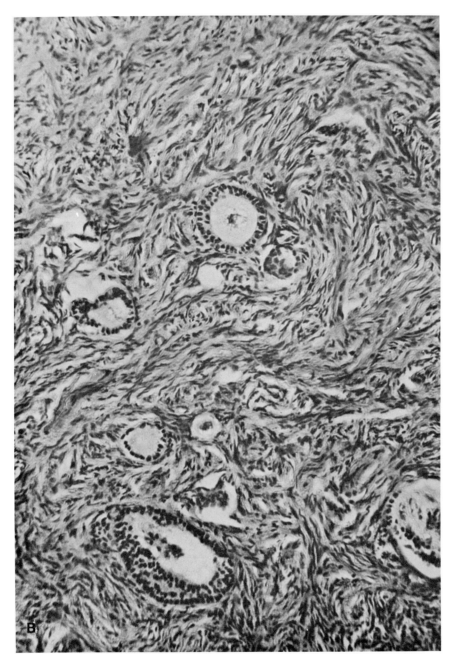

Laparotomy revealed hypoplastic dysgenetic ovaries with cortical remnants. Bilateral oophorectomy was done. Substitution therapy has promoted general well-being. Examination of ovarian sections (Fig. 6-4) showed fibrotic stroma, a thin cortex, and scanty fibrosed primordial follicles.

A sister, aged 21, had primary amenorrhea, an elevated FSH level and a 46 XX karyotype. Growth and development of the sisters were identical.

These patients had normal female chromosomal patterns, although some may have had other stemlines that would have proved mosaicism. Only blood cell cultures were performed. Deficient estrogen secretion was apparent. Each showed sex chromatin as well as elevated levels of FSH. Culdoscopy was possible in one of the first pair of sisters and revealed totally inactive and underdeveloped ovaries; oophorectomy in one of the second set of sisters also revealed underdeveloped ovaries.

The possibility of a genetic defect is suggested by the presence of the same abnormality in two sets of sisters. The existence of an autosomal recessive form of gonadal dysgenesis is suggested by Simpson and Christakos.[5]

A third group of patients with normal female karyotypes, 46 XX, experienced normal growth and development and menarche. After a few years, however, menstruation spontaneously stopped.

Primary ovarian failure, karyotype 46 XX. OCHS 419-575. A 26-year-old white female underwent normal growth and development with menarche at age 12. Her menses occurred at 4-week intervals until the age of 16 or 17, when menstruation spontaneously stopped. At that time her height was $63\frac{1}{2}$ in. Her weight had increased to a maximum of 134 lb 4 years before hospital admission. Treatment with thyroid failed to overcome her amenorrhea. She had failed to respond to one course of menopausal gonadotropins. Administration of ovarian replacement hormones, either as sequential therapy or as combined estrogen-progestogen medication produced withdrawal bleeding. She had no vasomotor symptoms and noted a decreased rate of growth of axillary hair.

Physical examination showed her height to be 64 in. and her weight $127\frac{3}{4}$ lb. Her breasts were normally developed. No secretion was noted. The vaginal mucosa was hypoestrogenic. Both cervix and uterus were infantile.

A Papanicolaou smear revealed the presence of sex chromatin. X-ray examination of the sella turcica disclosed no abnormality. Previous examinations elsewhere had indicated that 17-ketosteroid excretion was within normal limits. On one examination pituitary FSH was between 6 and 16 MU/24 hours, which was considered normal for that laboratory. A biopsy of the ovaries through the cul-de-sac in another institution revealed scanty primordial and atretic follicles in ovaries measuring 2 by 1 cm which were described as "inactive." Karyotype was normal female, 46 XX. The patient has been advised to continue ovarian replacement hormones.

Primary ovarian failure, karyotype 46 XX. OCHS 435-785. This 25-year-old white woman began menstruating at the age of 16. She had irregular menstrual periods until the age of 20. When she married at the age of 20, she began taking Ortho-Novum 2 for birth control, but stopped the ovarian suppressive agent after 6 months. She had no menses since that time. She was given clomiphene on two different occasions, without the induction of menses. One sister was normally fertile.

The patient's height was 61½ in. and her weight 94 lb. Her breasts were normally developed. The axillary and pubic hair was normally distributed. The vagina was normal and healthy. The maturation index was II. The cervix could be probed easily and the uterus was normal in size and movable. The adnexal zones were normal.

On two examinations the FSH was less than 6 MU/24 hours and between 16 and 50 MU/24 hours. 17-Ketosteroids were 5.5 mg/24 hours. Normal range in this laboratory is 5–15 mg/24 hours.

Both progesterone and human chorionic gonadotropins were administered, but failed to initiate menstrual bleeding. Her karyotype was 46 XX, with what was interpreted as a mild abnormality of the second X chromosome.

Menarche followed by cyclic menstruation and then cessation of menses after 1–10 years has been diagnosed as primary ovarian failure. These women have had brief periods of relatively normal cycles with spontaneously occurring amenorrhea generally unresponsive to large amounts of human menopausal gonadotropins.[1] The karyotype of such patients is usually 46 XX, but in rare instances mosaicism has been noted.

The etiology of primary ovarian failure is unknown, but a report by Netter and Sedaoun [4] suggests that an inadequate number of primordial follicles develops from a decreased number of germinal cells or gonocytes migrating to the ovarian cortex. Possibly there is an increase in the atretic process that destroys the primordial follicles.[1]

REFERENCES

1. DeMoraes-Ruehsen, M., and Jones, G. S. Premature ovarian failure. *Fertil Steril 18*:440, 1967.

2. JACOBS, P. A., HARNDEN, D. G., BUCKTON, K. E., BROWN, W. M., KING, M. J., McBRIDE, J. A., MACGREGOR, T. N., and MACLEAN, N. Cytogenic studies in primary amenorrhoea. *Lancet 1:*1183, 1961.
3. KADOTANI, T., OHAMA, K., and SATO, H. A preliminary cytogenetic survey in primary amenorrhea. *Jap J Hum Genet 13:*278, 1969. Abstracted in *Yearbook of Obstetrics and Gynecology,* 1970, p. 497.
4. NETTER, A., and SEDAOUN, M. Early menopause: Clinical, anatomic and chromosomal study of 16 cases, including 2 mosaics; relations to gonadal dysgenesis and the Stein-Leventhal syndrome. *Gynecol Obstet 66:*249, 1967. Abstracted in *Yearbook of Obstetrics and Gynecology,* 1968, p. 507.
5. SIMPSON, J. L., and CHRISTAKOS, A. C. Hereditary factors in obstetrics and gynecology. *Obstet Gynecol Surv 24:*580, 1969.
6. WILLIAMS, D. L., and RUNYAN, J. W. Sex chromatin and chromosome analysis in the diagnosis of sex abnormalities. *Ann Intern Med 64:*422, 1966.

Chapter Seven

Anomalies
of the Tubes

Cary M. Dougherty

The derivatives of the embryonic müllerian ducts in the female are, in the order of appearance, the fallopian tubes and the uterus. No instance has been reported of the absence of the tubes but presence of the uterus. The converse anomaly, presence of the tubes with absence of the uterus, has been observed and is possible because of the sequence of events in formation of the müllerian duct. The müllerian duct starts in the 11-mm embryo as a shallow, grooved depression near the cephalic pole of the wolffian body. Its cephalic end stays open, funnel-like, while its caudal end proliferates and tunnels backward along the route taken by the wolffian duct. The lateral margins of the groove incline toward each other, fuse, and enclose all but the open funnel in front. The "seam" formed by the fusion of the lips of the groove may not be tight and continuous, but may at first have irregular openings along its extent. Toward the tail end of the 32-mm embryo the duct curves medially and, meeting its contralateral partner, bends itself caudal again to continue the short distance to the wall of the urogenital sinus.

The observed abnormalities of the fallopian tubes and the uterus can be related almost mathematically to steps in the genesis and growth of the müllerian duct. Experience is limited by the rarity of tubal anomalies, but patterns are fairly definite.

AGENESIS OF THE FALLOPIAN TUBE

Absence of Both Tubes

In certain types of genital malformations the fallopian tubes are very small and inconspicuous and may not be noted at first inspection. Sometimes one side is without a tube while the other side possesses one. There are occasions, nevertheless, where the observation has been made by an experienced surgeon and substantiated by biopsy of the absence of both fallopian tubes. The condition is associated with absence of the uterus as well and usually with major abnormality of external and internal genital organs (e.g., testicular feminization).

Absence of One Tube

When the fallopian tube is not present on a side, half of the uterus (the part belonging to that side) does not develop either. The consequence is unicornuate uterus. The broad ligament is also likely to be incomplete or missing. Like bilateral absence, unilateral absence of the tube is found in association with defective gonadal development. The gonadal defect may also be one-sided.

Incomplete Tube

Sharply localized agenesis of one fallopian tube produces a defective ovum-transfer apparatus on one side (Fig. 3-36). Failure of development of the caudal portion of the tube is necessarily accompanied by failure of formation of the hemiuterus on the same side. The cranial segment of the tube may be completely normally developed. In one patient studied by us the tube was of such perfect proportions, except for the localized agenesis, that it could have been surgically engrafted into the unicornuate uterus.

Rudimentary Tube

There may be no more than a fibromuscular cord in the place of the tube, the epithelial lumen being absent. Such a rudimentary tube cannot be stimulated by hormones to function.

Infantile or Hypoplastic Tube

The fallopian tube in the infant and prepubertal female is a long, thin, almost cord-like structure. Although the several components (endosalpinx, myosalpinx, mesosalpinx, and fimbriated ostium abdominale) are hypoplastic, they are all present. When the tubes of an 18-year-old female are found at operation to be like those of an infant or child, they may be rightly called infantile, but not rudimentary. Under appropriate hormonal stimulation, infantile or hypoplastic tubes may be expected to undergo mature development. Whether they function depends upon the normality of the rest of the genital tract.

Etiology and Pathogenesis

Errors in development of the tube must begin at a time when the gonad is still in the indifferent stage. The müllerian duct follows after establishment of the wolffian body and duct. Thus, absence of the wolffian duct on one side would probably lead to absence of the müllerian duct and ultimately of the tube on that side. In addition, a kidney fault would result from the original wolffian duct fault.

After formation of the tube, its subsequent growth and development probably depend upon organizers from the ovary or absence of male organizers from the testis. When these substances are not functional in the normal manner, the tube is rudimentary or infantile instead of normal.

Diagnosis

There is no way of telling the exact state of formation and development of the fallopian tubes at clinical examination. Abnormality of the tube may be suspected in certain of the syndromes of gonadal anomaly. The condition is recognized at the time of surgical operation. Palpation of the free border of the broad ligament reveals whether there is a thin tube, a fibromuscular cord, or no extra tissue at all.

Differentiation from Wolffian Duct (Vas Deferens)

In individuals with incomplete sex differentiation, the surgeon may have to distinguish müllerian-derived from wolffian-derived ductal structures at the time of surgical operation. This can be done by determining where the tube begins and where it leads. The fallopian tube may be thought of as starting at the abdominal ostium and ending in the midline in relation to the uterine fundus; if that organ is missing the tube ends in a web of tissue far away from the bladder neck. The tube is a companion of a gonad which is expected to be ovary. The vas deferens begins at an epididymis attached to a gonad (abdominal or scrotal) and curves downward intraabdominally toward the base of the urinary bladder. The ductus deferens is of a smaller diameter than the fallopian tube. It does not have a mesentery, and it appears somewhat lighter colored.

Histologic examination allows definitive differentiation.

DUPLICATION OF OSTIUM

Careful inspection of the fimbriated end of the fallopian tube often reveals two openings, usually one larger than the other. A band of musculature separates them. The arrangement may be a main opening at the end with an accessory aperture on one side of the ampullary region.

The explanation of formation of two openings is straightforward. The müllerian funnel simply is duplicated or the edges of the groove failed to fuse completely.

ACCESSORY TUBE

It is not unusual to find one or several accessory fallopian tubes. Gardiner *et al.* have pointed out that the small cystic hydatids of Morgagni are formed from the müllerian funnel and are lined by müllerian epithelium and hence might be considered accessory tubes.[1] These same authors picture a histologic section showing a three-branched tube with three ostii abdominales.

We have seen several patients with a miniature tube complete with fimbriated end attached to the mesosalpinx. These small structures usually do not possess lumina and do not, therefore, have epithelial linings.

Pathogenesis

Since the müllerian funnel is not a simple dimple in the urogenital mass, but rather a frilly proliferation of the epithelium, the possibility exists that two grooved invaginations could begin at about the same time. This event would probably result from overactivity of the organizing mechanism, since the defect is not one which would be expected to have a genetic etiology. As far as is known, no animal has double müllerian ducts as standard equipment.

Treatment

None of the conditions described requires treatment apart from the management of other concomitant and more serious anomalies.

REFERENCE

1. GARDNER, G. H., GREENE, R. R., and PECKHAM, B. M. Solid and cystic structures of the broad ligament. *Am J Obstet Gynecol* 55:917, 1948.

Chapter Eight

Anomalies
of the Uterus

Cary M. Dougherty

Since the functions of the uterus are exclusively menstrual and reproductive, malfunctions caused by developmental defects would be expected to become apparent at puberty. Often however, uterine anomalies
are associated with other defects easily detected before the age of maturity. For example, maldevelopment of the uterus may be associated
with agenesis of the vagina.

No doubt there are instances where not a vestige of uterus, lining or
muscle, or even condensation of the supporting tissues is present. Such
a state would result if the müllerian ducts failed to grow caudally to the
position where the uterus is normally formed. A more likely abnormality is failure of the embryonic structures to mature into a "usable"
organ. In such cases vestigial cords of muscle are noted that do not contain an epithelial lumen. Case records often note divergent findings:
One examiner states the uterus is absent, while another describes two
rudimentary cords merging in the midline behind the urinary bladder
into a small but definite uterus. There are at least three degrees of
"absence" of the uterus, each having a somewhat different cause. They
are agenesis, vestigial müllerian remnants, and infantile or hypoplastic
uterus. The examiner must be careful to identify these conditions accurately in order to employ the proper treatment.

The uterus which is double in part or all of its extent may function

209

so well that its true anatomic architecture is never discovered. On the other hand, the defect may lead to a surgical emergency demanding operative correction. The surgeon must understand the abnormality confronting him so he can relieve the condition without doing unnecessary harm to distorted structures which will require later repair.

In describing developmental defects of the uterus, the following definitions are used. *Agenesis* is lack or absence of development; *aplasia* is incomplete or faulty development; *hypoplasia* is arrested development in which the uterus remains below the normal size or in an immature state. *Vestigial* means a condition of degenerate or imperfect development of the uterus which has been more normally developed in an earlier stage. *Rudimentary* uterus contains the basic elements in an initial state but no further refinements or differentiation into more mature elements. The *infantile* organ is the fully developed and formed but immature uterus of the normal infant. It is abnormal only if found in a mature woman.

MALDEVELOPMENT OF THE UTERUS

Absence

Detected only at time of surgical operation and then only if the surgeon is meticulous in his examination, absence is one of the rarest of uterine abnormalities. The ovaries may be "pieces of tissue resembling ovary" or they may be more or less completely normal even to the point of containing corpora lutea—incontrovertible evidence of normal function.

The tubes may appear normal in the greater portion of their length. The caudal ends of these tubes usually taper off within the supporting tissue of the broad ligament.

Vestigial Müllerian Remnants

This abnormality, like the preceding one, can be diagnosed only by surgical exploration of the pelvic cavity. Whereas absence of the uterus might mean that the müllerian duct did not grow all the way caudally to the urogenital sinus, in the condition under discussion the remnants indicate that these ducts did reach their destination. In the first case the müllerian ducts did not receive the growth stimulus; in the second they did not progress to organ formation. The vestiges are usually described as thin cords of fibromuscular tissue continuous with the fallopian tubes. Their course is medial and caudal, in some instances joining the opposite member of the pair in the midline; in other cases, remaining separate cords.

Rudimentary Uterus

In some cases the müllerian ducts form a structure which has the basic shape of uterus but which does not develop into that organ. The ducts may fuse in the midline, but develop no epithelial cavity. Each duct may form a rudimentary horn, fail in the fusing, and end in the fibromuscular tissue between the bladder and rectum. All possible combinations of smooth muscular wall and epithelial cavity have been observed. Often the body of the uterus may be recognized as an elongated ovoid mass in the midline. On occasion the surgeon removes a minute pear-shaped uterus only to be informed by the pathologist that there is no endometrial cavity or that the cavity occupies only a portion of the organ.

Connections with the Tubes

In most instances the surgeon is able to identify normal fallopian tubes with fimbriated ends. The caudal ends of the tubes either blend with the supportive tissues medially, "appear to be a part of the ovarian ligament," or continue medially and caudally as fibromuscular cords. In the unusual case of a rudimentary unicornuate uterus, there may be no tube on the opposite side.

Relation with the Ovary

In nearly every case the ovaries are intact even though the uterus is absent, vestigial, or rudimentary. Quite often the ovaries contain follicular cysts or actual corpora lutea, proof that they are competent sex glands with a reproductive capacity. When there is no uterus, the utero-ovarian ligament is not well formed, and often the round ligaments of the uterus do not appear normally developed. In these instances the ovaries are described as being suspended against the lateral pelvic wall or lodged at the internal inguinal ring. None of our patients had inguinal ovaries, however. In the sexually immature girl the ovaries appear as small but normally shaped organs attached along with the tubes to the free edge of the broad ligaments.

Connections with the Cervix and Vagina

When the uterus is absent, vestigial, or rudimentary the cervix is absent or vestigial. Sometimes the careful examiner may find a small thickened mass of tissue in the place where cervix should be located. In none of our patients was there a cervix with cervical canal at the apex of the vagina.

When the uterus and cervix are absent or vestigial, the vagina is nearly always rudimentary, varying from dimple-like to 4–5 cm in depth.

The diameter is usually much less than that of the normal organ. The urethra and vaginal vestibule are essentially normally formed and there is usually a hymen present, except in absence of the vagina.

Abnormalities of the Kidneys

Almost half the patients with agenesis of the uterus also have a major abnormality of the kidneys. These defects are pelvic kidney, horseshoe kidney, hypoplastic kidney, and agenesis of the kidney. Other defects of lesser degree undoubtedly occur, such as fetal lobulation, double calyx, and double ureter.

Stage at Which Defects Occur

The first of the three possible times at which developmental defects of the uterus may originate is at the 11-mm, 5-week stage, when the müllerian funnel first appears. If the müllerian duct is not formed both uterus and fallopian tubes will be absent. The second time at which anomalous development occurs is between inception of the müllerian duct and the time it reaches the urogenital sinus at 32 mm, 9 weeks. If development is arrested during this period, there will be only fallopian tubes formed or tubes with the vestiges of the ducts occupying the place where the uterus should have been located. If unilateral impairment takes place, the fault is unilateral absence of the tube with unicornuate uterus. In none of our specimens did the surgeon describe unicornuate uterus with partial tube formation on the side of the missing uterine horn, although this combination was found in one of the fetuses of the Spencer collection.

The third stage of development at which normal processes may go awry is that involving fusion of the müllerian ducts to form the uterus with condensation of mesenchyme about the genital canal forming a single organ in the midline—40–65 mm, 10–12 weeks. Failure of fusion may be complete or incomplete. It may result in production of any type of bicornuate or double uterus, and the resulting double uterus may condition the development of double vaginas (septate vagina). With failure of fusion there may be early regression of the müllerian ducts, leaving vestiges.

Infantile Uterus

Infantile uterus in the normal infant is not a defect. However, such a uterus in a postpubertal girl is anomalous. The uterus possesses a muscular corpus, a large fibrous cervix, and both endometrial and endocervical cavities lined by columnar epithelium. The distinguishing feature of the infantile uterus is its ability to respond to estrogen stimulation by maturing and achieving cyclic function.

There are two important practical clinical considerations in managing a patient with infantile uterus. First, administration of estrogens may, by promoting cyclic functioning, help her to feel more woman-like. Second, before initiating such treatment, the physician must ascertain that the infantile uterus is connected to an intact vaginal tract through which the menstrual discharge can find egress; otherwise, hematometra will result.

Treatment

With the exception of infantile uterus there is no treatment for any of the forms of maldevelopment described above. It is not necessary to remove a rudimentary or vestigial uterus unless it contains a partial or incomplete cavity which could interfere with hormonal treatment by forming an encysted hematoma. On the other hand, there is no contra-indication to removing such malformed organs if there is doubt about their structure.

Since abnormality of the vagina so often accompanies that of the uterus, plastic reconstruction of the vagina is often undertaken. A continuous channel for drainage of menstrual fluid is essential if a uterus is allowed to remain and if estrogens are used to stimulate genital tissues and organs.

UTERUS UNICORNIS

Only four case histories are on record at Charity Hospital of patients with unicornuate uterus.[15] This infrequency may be due in part to the difficulty of recognizing the patient with the defect. There may be no impairment of reproductive ability—our patients all conceived and carried their babies to term, and the findings on clinical examination are not distinctively different from the normal. The accidental discovery of the unsuspected condition is the rule in most instances.

Uterus

The unicornuate uterus is about the same size as the normally formed organ but is asymmetrical, with the fundus inclining and tapering toward the side with the fallopian tube. Only one round ligament is present, that on the same side as the tube. The opposite side of the fundus is smoothly rounded with no attachments. The broad ligament is altered or absent, and there is evidence that the blood supply including the uterine artery may be anomalous also. Although not always mentioned in reports, the uterosacral ligaments are probably usually both present. Peritoneal reflections from the unicornuate uterus ventrally and dorsally are like those of the normal uterus, but on the side of the missing horn the reflection is, of course, considerably lower.

Findings in other types of uterine maldevelopment suggest that the uterine vessels may be anomalous, branched, or rudimentary on the side of the deformity.

Endometrial Cavity

The endometrial cavity of the unicornuate uterus is shaped differently from and may be smaller than that of the normal uterus. When viewed from the front it is long and ovoid, with ends tapered toward the cornu and the endocervix.

Ovary

The ovary on the same side as the single-horned uterus is normally formed and functional. Mesovarium, suspensory ligament, and utero-ovarian ligament are intact and in correct relation with the respective organs. The ovary on the opposite side may be absent (as in our patients), suspended against the lateral pelvic wall, or held close to the internal inguinal ring. When present it is apt to be functional.

Fallopian Tubes

The fallopian tube on the side of the uterine horn is normal, complete with fimbriated abdominal ostium and mesosalpinx. Its insertion into the fundus of the uterus may appear slightly different, since the fundus does not have the usual convexity and bilateral symmetry. The fallopian tube opposite the horn may be absent (as in our patients) or may be represented by a vestigial remnant or cord-like structure which does not form a part of the uterus. There may be a hypoplastic or even a normal cranial (inner, abdominal) segment of tube which does not join the uterus. If the tube is present there is also formed at least some part of the broad ligament. When the tube is absent the broad ligament is also not developed.

Cervix and Vagina

The portio vaginalis, os, and canal of the cervix of the unicornuate uterus are not appreciably different from those of the cervix of the normal uterus. There is no possibility of formation of double cervices in the true unicornuate uterus. The cervix may be somewhat smaller than average for the normal organ, but is not necessarily so. Double vaginas are not found in conjunction with the unicornuate uterine deformity.

Urinary System

Malformations and absence of some parts of the urinary system are common associates of this genital abnormality. Absence of the kidney on the side of the defect may be noted (as in our patients).

Pathogenesis

A unicornuate uterus is formed when only one of the pair of müllerian ducts grows down to the urogenital sinus. The aberrant duct may be missing altogether, or it may be present in only its cranial extent. When it is missing completely the wolffian duct also is probably defective or absent, since it is developed first and appears to act as a guide for the course of the müllerian duct. When ovary, tube, and one horn of the uterus are all missing (as in our patients), the cause may be failure of development of the entire urogenital ridge including mesonephric, gonadal, and ductal portions. When part of the urinary system, e.g., one kidney, is absent along with part of the genital ductal apparatus, the original fault lies with the wolffian duct.

Treatment

There is little opportunity, and often no reason, to try to improve the unicornuate uterus. The patient should be given a detailed explanation of her unusual anatomy and be advised to live with it, since it does not lead to life-threatening sequelae.

DUPLICATION OF THE UTERUS

Uterus didelphys and uterus bicornis are well-known but rather unusual malformations of the uterus stemming from failure of unification or partial unification of the müllerian ducts. The following discussion is based on a review of the records of 74 patients with various types of uterine duplication. Several characteristics in the records of these cases are notable: diagnosis was not easy, often arrived at by chance; certain diagnostic errors were made again and again as new house staff physicians encountered the same problems as their predecessors and followed the same false trails rather than learning by precept; and certain combinations of malformations seemed to be present together in the same patient.

Types of Double Uterus

There are many degrees and types of duplication, some involving extensive and some minor alteration. Our review, which was retrospective, did not permit such fine discrimination. We classified our patients into four categories only: *uterus didelphys, uterus bicornis unicollis, uterus bicornis with rudimentary horn,* and *rudimentary bicornuate uterus* (Fig. 8-1). It would have been desirable clinically to distinguish the *septate uterus,* but this could not be done in our study. A few exceptional cases were recorded in great detail and afforded opportunity for observations upon the more unusual malformations.

Pathogenesis

The several degrees and types of duplication of the uterus are caused by the same basic fault: failure of fusion of the paired müllerian ducts in the caudal region where they lie in apposition. Anomaly of the wolffian duct may be primarily at fault when there is associated renal agenesis. In such cases the failure of the wolffian duct to extend far enough caudally may be the responsible factor. In this regard, it is curious that in all seven patients with unilateral renal agenesis the defect was on the right side. The reason for this is obscure.

When both müllerian ducts develop their full length and reach caudally to the urogenital sinus, they must not only fuse along the total extent of the part called uterovaginal or primitive genital canal but participate with the sinus epithelium in forming the vaginal cord. Thus, unfused "uterine" portions would lead either to the persistence of a septum of the uterus or to actual duplication of the body or entire uterus, while unfused caudal portions would lead to formation of two vaginas as well. It has been noted by a number of investigators that fusion of the müllerian ducts takes place by dissolution of the intervening duct walls from a caudal to cranial direction. It is, accordingly, possible for a patient to have one cervix and two corpora but never one corpus and two cervices or one cervix and uterus with two vaginas.

Comparative Anatomy

It has been suggested that the double uterus is probably not a defect or malformation but an atavism, since it can be seen in its several different manifestations in the lower animals. Jarcho summarized these aspects of the anatomy of the uterus by noting "in mammals, starting with the lower species, all the theoretical intermediate evolutionary stages have their counterpart in humans, ranging from double uterus to single uterus. Thus . . . monotremes have two separate uteri without vaginae, whereas marsupials have two separate uteri with separate vaginae. Among placental mammals a double uterus is found in certain rodents, bats, and the aardvark. A beginning of fusion between the two uteri is evident in pigs, cattle, certain rodents, certain bats, and carnivores. A two-horned uterus is characteristic of ungulates, cetaceans, in-

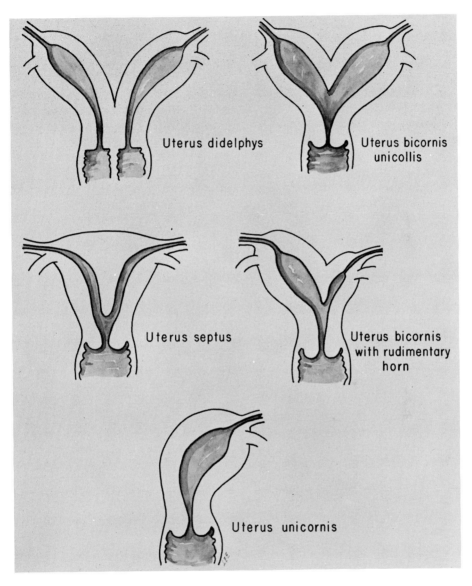

Fig. 8-1. Different forms of anomalous uteri.

sectivores, and some carnivores, while a single uterus, the uterus simplex, is found in apes and humans." [8]

Uterus Didelphys

Definition

This term is used to identify the organ with separate cavities and cervices. Most of the specimens also have separate uterine bodies, i.e., they present the bicornuate form when examined intraabdominally, and the two are joined in the region of the cervix. This anomaly is also called *uterus bicornis bicollis.* Technically, the term may not be correct in all cases, since the uterine horns may be fused even though the cavities are separate. The uterus having a complete septum continuous to the external cervical os or continuous with a vaginal partition may be classified as a form of uterus didelphys. The management of a patient with such a uterus depends upon the thickness of the septum and the ease with which it can be divided from the vaginal approach. All degrees of thickness or thinness have been observed.

Uterus

At laparotomy the surgeon usually finds two more or less distinct horns separated by a deep cleft. Each horn is slightly smaller than the normal uterus, and the two are symmetrical, one a mirror image of the other. The double uterus with asymmetrical horns has been described also (bicornuate uterus with rudimentary horn), but it is the exception rather than the rule. Fusion of the myometrium of the horns into one muscular body represents another exceptional shape. In these specimens the two uterine cavities remain apart. Many of our records describe a midsagittal fold, veil, or band of peritoneum extending from the bladder in front to the rectum behind and passing through the notch between the uterine horns. An embryologic explanation for this structure is not apparent. It may be a remnant of the caudal portion of the ventral mesentery of the gut.

The peritoneal reflection on the anterior (ventral) aspect of the double uterus is lower than on the normal uterus. The fold is possibly displaced down by the intercornual fissure, for when the uterine musculature is fused into a single external form, the peritoneal plica stretches from one side to the other just below the attachments of the round ligaments in a manner comparable to the normal. The posterior cul-de-sac (pouch of Douglas) is well formed, and one uterosacral ligament attaches to each cervix. At the opposite extremity of the organ a single round ligament is inserted into the myometrium just below the apex of each horn. This ligament may be attenuated or more or less normal in size.

Circulatory apparatus of the double uterus is probably usually normal; no anomalies were recognized in our patients. Arteriography done on one parous patient (BR-196237) showed normal uterine arteries bilaterally.

Each cavity of the uterus didelphys is smaller than the one cavity of the normal uterus. The combined surface area of the two, however, is greater than the endometrial surfaces of the single organ. By means of x-ray the cavities can be seen as long ovals with ends pointed at the tubal attachment and the endocervical canal. Since the cavities are not connected, there is less available space for expansion during gestation in either one than in the normally united uterus.

Tubes and Ovaries

A fallopian tube is attached to each horn of the double uterus at its apex, which tends to be conical rather than rounded. The relation with the round ligament is the same as in the normal uterus. The tube is of usual diameter and length. The ovaries are described as being of the normal size and appearance. They are attached, each to a uterine horn on the respective side, by the utero-ovarian ligament in the normal manner.

Cervix and Vagina

By definition uterus didelphys is double uterus complete with a cervix for each uterine corpus. The double cervices are not exactly like two single cervices, however. On vaginal speculum examination they are seen to be bilaterally symmetrical but partly flattened and strongly attached to each other in the midline by fusion of their fibrous tissue bodies. They do not usually protrude into the upper vagina in the manner of the normal portio vaginalis of the single cervix but form instead a double doughnut-shaped portio vaginalis. The external os and canal of the cervices are patent and of a size sufficient to function in both conception and parturition. Upon occasion the two cervices may not be the same size, one being well formed and the other hypoplastic. There may be one oversized cervix with a thin partition dividing the canal into two separate spaces.

When examined vaginally all but 1 of our 22 patients with uterus didelphys had double vaginas. In some of the multiparous patients the septum had been disrupted, presumably by vaginal delivery. In the typical case the septum extends to the hymenal ring, forming at the introitus a septate hymen. The septum may be quite thin but is usually about the same thickness as the other parts of the vaginal wall. A definite component of fibromuscular supporting tissue can be identified.

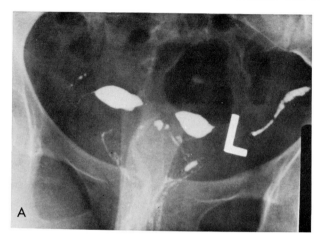

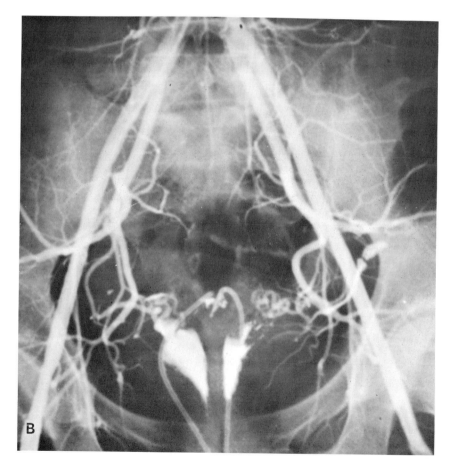

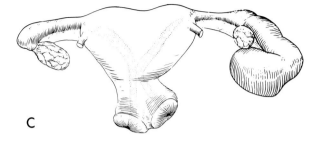

Fig. 8-2. Uterus didelphys with fused cornua. BR-196237. *A*. Hysterosalpingo-gram. *B*. Pelvic arteriogram. Polyethylene tubes within uterine cavities show tortuous arteries of normal size. *C*. Endometrial cavities are separate, each having a cervical opening.

Each of the two vaginas is somewhat smaller in diameter than the normal single vagina, though not too small for coitus. One of our patients (BR-196237) volunteered the information that intercourse was possible and feasible in both organs, and both members of the couple requested that the septum be left intact.

Uterus didephys with single corpus. BR-196237. (Patient of Dr. Brooks Cronan, Baton Rouge.) This 30-year-old white female, para 2, complained of excessive menstrual flow. She had had no trouble becoming pregnant, but could not deliver vaginally because of malpresentation of the fetuses. She had been told that she had two vaginas and two cervices. When the patient was examined the doctor noted that she had a septate vagina with the septum extending from hymen to the cervix. The vaginas were of equal size. There was a cervical portio vaginalis at the apex of each vagina. The vaginal septum was continuous with the partition which separated the two cervices. Both cervical canals were patent. Preoperative studies consisted of utero-salpingography, pelvic arteriography, and pyelography. Uterine cavities were separate, fallopian tubes were patent to distal ends which were closed, and kidney pelves were normal (Fig. 8-2*A*).

Uterine arteries were demonstrated and seemed to be of ample caliber (Fig. 8-2*B*).

The uterus, tubes, and ovaries were removed by laparotomy. It was seen that the uterine body was single but larger than the normal organ while both tubes presented the appearance of hydrosalpinx (Fig. 8-2*C*).

The ovaries were bound to the tubes with dense fibrous adhesions.

All the uterine ligaments were of normal appearance and were attached at the proper location.

When there are two cervices there are almost always two equal-sized vaginas, one for each cervix and uterus. Occasionally one vagina is smaller or ends in a blind pouch, or there is a transverse septum. Hematometrocolpos was formed in one of our patients.

In the usual case the vaginal septum extends from hymen to the midline between cervices, but the septum may be incomplete in the region of the cervical ora. A diagnostic problem in this case is to determine whether there are actually two cervices. We found notations on many records that one examiner described a single cervix while another examiner found two. One case history (CH62-3763) details an argument between two residents who saw a patient on alternate visits to the clinic: One resident maintained there was a single cervix, the other identified two. The argument was settled when one of the residents painted "the cervix" with Schiller's stain and then exposed another one which was unstained.

Urinary Tract Anomalies

Among 14 patients with uterus didelphys studied by pyelography, 2 had agenesis of the right kidney and 1 had duplication of the right kidney pelvis. Bilateral renal agenesis has been thoroughly studied and the relation of this major defect to anomalies of the müllerian system has been noted.[3,7] The high incidence of urinary tract anomalies among women with genital defects has long attracted attention.[11]

Uterus Bicornis Unicollis

Definition

The uterus with two-horned external configuration is, strictly speaking, a *bicornuate uterus*. If it also possesses a single cervix the term *unicollis* applies. The uterine cavity and endocervical canal together make up a Y-shaped space, easily demonstrated by x-ray examination without resort to surgical exploration of the pelvic cavity. Often, however, x-rays demonstrate the Y-shaped cavity, but surgical exploration proves the uterus to have only a single muscular body or at most only a shallow notch in the fundus. This anomaly has been called *septate uterus* and classified separately from bicornuate uterus. Definitive classification is difficult if not impossible when x-ray examination shows a Y-shaped cavity but the patient refuses surgery, and when curettage discloses a partitioned uterus but neither x-ray nor surgical examination is available. Since these unproved cases cannot be disregarded in a study of the incidence of the anomaly, they are classified as bicornuate uterus of unspecified type.

Uterus

When inspected at the time of surgical operation, the body of the uterus bicornis unicollis presents a bifid configuration. It is misleading to try to judge the condition of the cervix, single or double, by the depth of the notch between the uterine horns, but in general a deep notch indicates duplication all the way while a shallow notch means duplication of the upper portion of the uterus with single cervix. As already noted the body of the uterus may not be two-horned, but possess only a crease across the fundus from front to back. This deformity is referred to in medical writing as *arcuate* uterus. The condition of the cavity, however, and not the external configuration determines the functional incapacity caused by anomalous development.

When there are two horns the attachments of the peritoneal folds and the ligaments are the same as in complete duplication, uterus didelphys. A single round ligament is attached to each cornu just below the junction of the tube. Often, a fold or band of peritoneum passes through the space between the horns from bladder to sigmoid. Palpation of the lower segment of the uterus and of the cervix through the adjacent structures will aid in determining the shape of the cervix and whether it is double.

When the horns of the uterus bicornis unicollis are symmetrical the uterine vessels are, in all probability, normally developed. Nevertheless, the possibility of defective vasculature should be considered when the function of the deformed uterus is evaluated.

The endometrial cavities of the two horns join in the region of the lower segment to form one with the endocervical canal. Therefore, in the aggregate there is more space lined by endometrium than is found in the normal uterus, but it is not as satisfactory for maintaining gestation because the ordinarily capacious fundus is partitioned.

Tubes and Ovaries

A normally formed tube is attached at the summit of each uterine horn. The mesosalpinx and abdominal end of the tube are not affected by the maldevelopment of the uterus. Ovaries are bilaterally present and appear completely normal. Ovarian function is indicated by the fact that it is usual for these patients to menstruate and to become pregnant.

Cervix and Vagina

On pelvic examination the cervix of the uterus bicornis unicollis is indistinguishable from the cervix of the normally formed uterus. A prominent portio vaginalis with external os and endocervical canal are found. An extreme variant of this type abnormality is the uterus with a thin septum which descends all the way to the external cervical os. Such a condition might be considered uterus didelphys.

In most cases the vagina is single, with fully developed hymen and fornices. Among some 30 patients at Charity Hospital, however, 3 had double vaginas, I had a partial vaginal septum, and I had agenesis of the vagina. The complete septum begins at the hymen and ends just in front of (caudal to) the cervix. The incomplete septum is found at either extremity of the vagina.

Urinary Tract Anomalies

Pyelography in 17 patients with bicornuate uterus proved agenesis of right kidney in 5 and probable absence of the left kidney in 1 patient. Doubtless there were lesser degrees of abnormality in other patients.

Uterus Bicornis with Rudimentary Horn

When the two horns of the bicornuate uterus are obviously asymmetrical, the anomaly may cause more trouble than when the horns are of equal size and possess complete endometrial cavities. The smaller of the two horns is anatomically and functionally imperfect. Clinical features may be distinctly different from those found in the symmetrical bicornuate uterus.

Uterus

Inspection of the uterus is possible only at surgical operation. Pelvic examination may indicate the presence of the abnormality, but hysterography is not reliable since the picture may suggest uterus unicornis. A single horn with one tube and one round ligament attached forms the main portion of the uterus. The rudimentary horn is much smaller. It may be attached low, near the cervical region, or higher, near the fundal portion. It may seem to arise from the point of attachment of the fallopian tube, and may appear more like an enlarged tube than a uterine horn. One surgeon described an "accessory fundus" at operation for pregnancy in a rudimentary uterine horn.

The major source of trouble is in the failure of the cavity of the small horn to connect with and drain into the cavity of the large horn or the cervical canal. If the rudimentary horn does not have a cavity, no special problems arise. If it has a small cavity lined by uterine mucosa, open at the tubal end but closed at the point where it should connect with the other cavity, hematometra or, in the event of implantation of an ovum within the small horn, an essentially ectopic pregnancy may occur. In

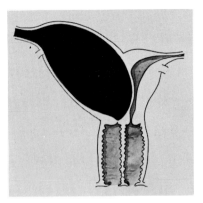

Fig. 8-3. Diagram of relations in case of right hematometra in uterus didelphys. CH56-222016.

the latter event the pregnancy must either rupture the small horn or be terminated by surgical operation.

Uterus didelphys with hematometra and right renal agenesis. CH56-222016. This 24-year-old white woman was admitted to the hospital for lower abdominal pain. She had undergone laparotomy 4 years earlier for removal of a large right-sided cystic mass which proved to be encysted blood within one horn of a double uterus, a condition brought about by atresia of the right cervix (Fig. 8-3). Two years following the first operation she had had surgical removal of the right cervical stump and vaginal septum.

Diagnostic procedures including x-ray, pyelography, and hysterography disclosed that the patient's right kidney was absent and that her left uterine tube was probably not patent. Palliative treatment alleviated her symptoms, but in time she sought consultation elsewhere which resulted in surgical removal of the remaining pelvic organs.

An interesting finding which may have resulted from the defective development of the genital tract was the presence of mucous columnar epithelium in large areas of the vagina.

It has been pointed out by Rolen *et al.*[12] that the uterine artery is anomalous on the side of the rudimentary horn, making the horn even less capable of supporting gestation.

Ovaries and Tubes

The ovaries are apparently normal in the recorded instances. Pregnancy in the rudimentary horn has been observed often enough to indicate that the ovary probably ovulates with average regularity.

The fallopian tubes are also normal, connecting with the horns on the respective sides. Their patency and confluence with the uterus is the rule, as proved by the frequency with which pregnancy in the rudimentary horn has been reported.[12]

Cervix and Vagina

There is one cervix. On pelvic examination the appearance is not distinctively different from the normal. Sounding of the cervix and endometrial cavity usually gives no additional information about the anomaly, since in most cases a connection with the cavity of the rudimentary horn cannot be found.

The vagina is single in most patients. No abnormality was noted in the 4 cases seen at Charity Hospital. Double vagina is possible, however, since the defect is essentially uterus bicornis unicollis.

Urinary Tract Abnormalities

Associated anomalies are noted with this defect as with other types of uterine duplication. Lobulation of the contralateral kidney was noted in one of our patients. Rolen *et al.* counted 15 published case histories, including 4 of their own, of bicornuate uterus with rudimentary horn studied by pyelography. Of the 15 patients 3 had normal upper urinary tracts, 10 had agenesis of the kidney on the side of the uterine defect, and 2 had pelvic kidneys on the same side.

Rudimentary Bicornuate Uterus

When exploratory laparotomy discloses an empty space in the pelvic region where the uterus should be, the first appraisal is that the uterus is absent. Careful examination may show, however, that in place of the uterus there are two fibrous cords, continuations of the fallopian tubes, which course toward the midline, turn caudalward, and enter the space between bladder and rectum. The cords do not contain lumina or epithelial components, and hence are vestigial remnants of the former müllerian ducts which failed to unite or form a uterus. The proper term for this condition is *vestigial müllerian ducts,* as they undoubtedly reached a further stage of development and then regressed. This type of "uterus" is always associated with vaginal agenesis. The combination of vestigial müllerian remnants and vaginal agenesis is sometimes encountered when the primary defect is gonadal or ovarian agenesis. This condition is discussed above in connection with uterine agenesis.

A small but definite uterus composed of two rudimentary horns may theoretically result from the same cause as the asymmetrical bicornuate uterus, differing only in that the causative factor is bilateral. Such a situation has not been encountered in the Charity Hospital records or in our own consultation cases.

Clinical Features of Double Uterus

Our study of the records of all types of double uterus disclosed no significant differences in clinical features among the several types. There may be differences between the most abnormal (uterus didelphys) and the least abnormal (uterus subseptus) forms of duplication, but such a comparison was not available to us. From our review we were able to arrive at a composite clinical picture as well as to note exceptional features.

Signs and Symptoms

Most instances of double uterus are found by routine examination or investigation of a decidedly minor symptom. The routines by which the impression is gained are vaginal speculum and bimanual pelvic examination, sounding of the uterine cavity, curettage of the endometrium, and hysterography.

The bicornuate uterus is sometimes discovered at the time of surgical operation for another condition, e.g., hematometra due to atresia of the lower genital tract or suspected myoma or ovarian tumor that is really one horn of a double uterus.

Complaints which may be related to the double uterus include abdominal pain, dyspareunia, dysmenorrhea, lower back pain, excessive bleeding at menstruation, sterility, repeated abortion, premature labor, malposition and malpresentation of fetus, and antenatal bleeding.

Hysterography

The most informative single procedure in the diagnostic work-up of the patient with anomalous uterus is x-ray visualization of the uterus and tubes; this must be done in every case. In order to learn position and relations of the two horns, oblique views as well as the anteroposterior view must be taken. At least one exposure should be made while the surgeon exerts traction on the cervix. We prefer to use a water-soluble rather than an oil-base contrast medium if laparotomy is not planned immediately. The pictures show various shapes of the rabbit-ears arrangement of the double cavities. They tend to come to points at the tubal ends, where the thread-like outlines of the tubal canals extend outward. The partition between the two cavities, be it partial or complete, does not possess perforations or intercommunications. In one of our patients (BRG 34411) such a defect of the septum did exist at the time of hysterography, but was the result of two cesarean section operations with transverse incisions in the lower segment of a uterus didelphys containing separate cavities and cervices but only one (fused) body.

It is imperative to visualize the kidneys and ureters. We have found it useful to combine pyelography with pelvic arteriography. Both can be accomplished in a single procedure by cannulating the femoral artery on one side to inject contrast medium. Immediate exposures demonstrate the uterine vessels while delayed films show the excretory organs. Information concerning both these sets of important structures is essential in planning proper treatment.

Contrast roentgenography after intraperitoneal injection of carbon dioxide (pneumogynecography) may be used to determine the configuration of the body of the uterus. There must be a limit, however, to the number of different diagnostic procedures done upon the same patient, and pneumogynecography need be done only when there are special considerations in management.

Septate uterus causing four spontaneous abortions. (Patient of Dr. Truman Hawes, Lafayette). This 27-year-old Caucasian consulted a gynecologist after having four spontaneous abortions, following the last of which she had curettage of the endometrial cavity. The referring physician found that she had bicornuate uterus, demonstrated by means of hysterography.

The gynecologist noted that the vagina and cervix were of completely normal appearance. Hysterosalpingography and pneumogynecography demonstrated that the uterus possessed two cavities joining a single endocervical canal and contained in a single muscular corpus. The shadows of the two uterine cavities formed a V-shaped design on the x-ray films (Fig. 8-4).

Surgical operation was carried out to remove the uterine septum. The surgeon noted that the uterus had no external markings to indicate that it contained two cavities. Both tubes and ovaries were completely normal to inspection. The two round ligaments were attached at the respective uterine cornua.

Menstrual Performance

The menstrual history of the patient with uterus bicornis may not be substantially different from normal. Relatively few patients have too heavy a flow, and other irregularities such as unequal cycles and cramps seem to be no more frequent than in normal women. Although the female with two endometrial cavities would be expected to have a greater than normal volume of bleeding, this does not seem to be the case, and many women with double uterus have no more blood loss than the average of normal women.

Fertility

There was no impairment of fertility among our patients. The percentage of nulligravida was somewhat lower than in the general population (slightly less than 1:3, nulliparous to parous). This observation is to be expected since the abnormality does not affect the ovaries, and the genital tract is patent and intact.

Obstetric Performance

The woman with bicornuate uterus experiences difficulty in carrying the conceptus to term and delivering a viable infant.[8,13] Almost one-third of all conceptions are *aborted spontaneously,* most in the first trimester. A third to a fourth of the remaining pregnancies end in premature delivery. About one-half or slightly more of the total pregnancies continue to term and produce a living child.

Uterus didelphys with fair obstetrical performance. CH49-355831. This 20-year-old Caucasian consulted a clinic physician for dysmenorrhea. She had had one early spontaneous abortion. Gynecologic examination disclosed two vaginas and two cervices. Hysterography showed two uterine cavities. The vaginal septum but not that of the uterus, was incised. In time the patient became pregnant six times; two pregnancies ended with early spontaneous abortion and four resulted in the birth of four living babies.

Uterus didelphys and double vagina, septum ruptured by vaginal delivery. CH55-169087. This 29-year-old Caucasian was seen on the obstetric unit with antenatal hemorrhage at 32 weeks' gestation. When the obstetrician performed a sterile vaginal examination he found a large sagittal tag of tissue attached along the anterior vaginal wall. Another similar ridge of tissue was seen on the midposterior wall. There were two cervices.

At cesarean section operation, the obstetrician described the uterus as having two horns, the small-sized baby occupying the larger horn. No reparative or other surgical measures were carried out.

At 6-weeks' check-up the finding of previously double vagina and bicornuate uterus were confirmed. It appeared that the vaginal septum had been ruptured in one of the five previous vaginal deliveries, and had healed satisfactorily leaving midsagittal ridges along the vagina.

Malpresentation of the fetus is found more often than in the normal gravida. *Breech presentation* is encountered most often of the abnormal lies, occurring at possibly two or three times the expected 3–4 per cent rate for breech delivery in the normal woman.

Sometimes the patient examined in advanced labor is found to have the baby presenting by breech with one buttock or lower extremity on either side of an incomplete vaginal septum. *Transverse presentation of*

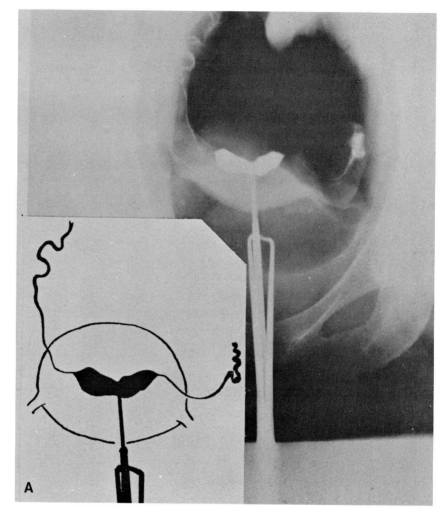

Fig. 8-4. Bicornuate uterus. *A.* Hysterosalpingogram and air-contrast x-ray. Angle of view is from above downward. *B.* X-ray from frontal angle shows two cavities and one cervix. V-shaped position of cavities, which form an acute angle, indicates that external contour of the uterus is one of a single corpus.

the fetus is also more common. Bizarre arrangement of the fetus may exist, the head and upper trunk situated in one uterine cornu while the lower trunk and extremities are in the other cornu. For good reason the babies thus presenting abnormally resist efforts at external version to a correct position.

Cesarean delivery is frequently necessary, not only for the abnormal

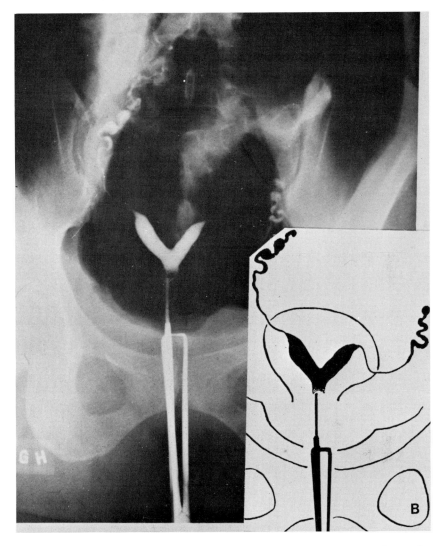

presentations but for failure of labor to progress. In some patients the firm, *fibrotic cervix* is at fault,[4] while in others *dysrhythmic contractions* of the myometrium prevent progress. Medical authors have mentioned obstruction of progress of labor by *incarceration* of the *second uterine horn.*[8] This consideration seems to be of more theoretical than actual importance.

In addition to the higher rate of dystocia in gravidas with double uterus, there are other obstetric complications. A higher rate of *stillbirths* can be anticipated. *Retained placenta* in the third stage is more common.

Not the least of the complications is *laceration* of the *lower genital tract,* cervix, vagina, and vaginal septum. Laceration of the vaginal septum does not always cause serious hemorrhage, however. A multiparous patient seen for the first time by an obstetrician may be found to have a healed laceration of the septum sustained in an earlier delivery attended by a midwife. That the lacerated septum healed without exsanguinating hemorrhage is evidence enough that the vascularity of the septum is not always great.

It has been suggested that unexplained vaginal bleeding during pregnancy may come from the nonpregnant horn of a double uterus. Older medical writers thought the nonpregnant uterine horn might continue to undergo cyclic change.[1] Such thinking conflicts with basic concepts of female endocrinology. When pregnancy occurs in one side, the mucosa in the other side undergoes the changes dictated by the hormonal milieu, i.e., it too produces the endometrium of pregnancy with stromal decidual reaction. This type of mucosa is maintained in the nonpregnant as well as the pregnant horn until termination of the pregnancy or until a change occurs in the hormonal pattern leading to termination of the pregnancy.

Superfetation has also been attributed to separate functions of two horns of the uterus.[6] Since the basic requirement for superfetation is compound ovulation rather than compound gestation space, an extra uterus or uterine horn would not suffice.

Simultaneous pregnancy in the two uterine horns has been reported.[2] Twin pregnancies also have occurred in one horn or in a rudimentary horn of a bicornuate uterus. The fact that the uterus may be bipartite probably does not alter the natural chance occurrence of twinning. Simultaneous pregnancies in each member of a uterus didelphys would be exceedingly rare, and there is no published report of such a case.

Pregnancy in a Rudimentary Horn

Since a rudimentary horn is much smaller than the normal uterus and does not connect with the main endometrial cavity, pregnancy within such a horn is not normal; it is, indeed, ectopic. Since the lumen of the horn is not always continuous with the lower genital tract, conception and implantation on that side can occur only by transabdominal migration of the sperm or of both sperm and ovum. An essential condition is the patency and normal functioning of the fallopian tube on the affected side.

In a review of 70 published case reports Rolen *et al.*[12] found that very few of the pregnancies progressed to fetal viability. The outcome was either rupture of the uterine horn in the first or second trimester, or fetal death forming an entrapped missed abortion. In either case, the only satisfactory means of termination would be surgical operation. Rupture of the gravid uterine horn is, of course, a grave surgical emergency. Hematoperitoneum, shock, and pain are part of the clinical findings.

Septate Uterus

There are certain special considerations if the double uterus is septate or partially septate. These are the least degrees of the abnormality and the clinical features are the least divergent from the normal. When clinical signs lead to the diagnosis of septate uterus, surgical correction entails a different principle of operation than that used in uniting two uterine horns.

Treatment of Double Uterus

Surgical correction of double uterus is indicated when abnormal menstrual or reproductive function results from the defect. The mere finding of an anomalous uterus is not in itself reason for operation, for the organ is often adequate for its purpose. In order of frequency of occurrence the indications for surgical intervention are abortion and prematurity, sterility, and menstrual disorders. The surgeon must know exactly the condition of the uterus before he sets out to reshape it surgically.

Uterus Didelphys

Surgical unification of the totally double uterus is not necessary in every case and is technically difficult or impossible when the two cervices are separately formed with heavy fibrous tissue. The extent of the surgical trauma—from fundus uteri to vaginal introitus—renders surgical operation not feasible in many cases. When the cervical septum is thin and the combined diameter of the canals not too large when joined, incision of the lower part of the partition from below may be part of the surgical unification of the uterus. In uniting the two horns of the selected uterus didelphys, the surgical operation popularized by Strassman is used.

Other surgical procedures of value in improving function are those to relieve cervical stenosis or atresia, remove vaginal stenosis caused by bands or septa, and to remedy obstetric complications. Hemihysterectomy serves no useful purpose and dissection of one cervix from the other is not practical.

Uterus Bicornis Unicollis

This type of deformity lends itself to surgical repair by the procedure of Strassman.[14] Preconditions of successful repair are that the horns are of approximately the same size and both contain an endometrial cavity

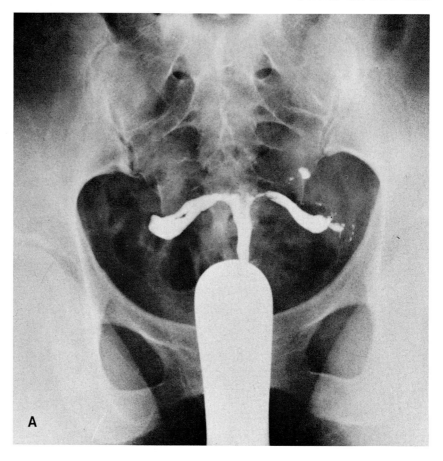

Fig. 8-5. Uterus bicornis unicollis. *A.* Hysterosalpingogram. Drooping appearance of two uterine cavities indicates body of uterus is formed into separate
horns. *B.* Pelvic arteriogram shows normal uterine arteries with adequate
blood supply.

connected with the cervix. This information is readily ascertained by
hysterography. The best results may be expected in the repair of uterus
bicornis unicollis.

Uterus bicornis unicollis corrected by metroplasty. (Patient of Dr. L. J.
Mickey, Monroe.) This 24-year-old Caucasian female had never been
pregnant. She consulted a gynecologist because, since her husband was
sterile, the couple wished her to have artificial insemination. Pelvic
examination disclosed normal vestibule, vagina and cervix. The uterus
was not clearly palpable and hysterosalpingography showed the uterus

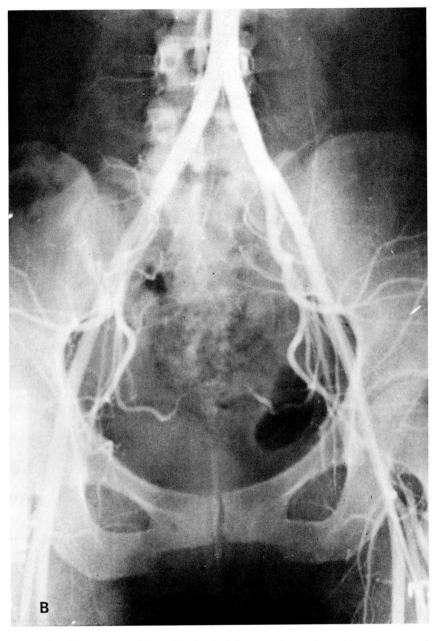

to be bicornuate (Fig. 8-5*A*). Pelvic arteriography showed normal uterine blood supply (Fig. 8-5*B*). The gynecologist recommended plastic unification of the uterus before artificial insemination.

Operation disclosed two uterine horns completely separated down

to the region of the internal cervical os. The transverse incision recommended by Strassman was made, and the two horns of the uterus
were sutured with interrupted stitches forming a uterine body which
was the size of the average normal uterus. Healing was satisfactory as
determined by follow-up hysterosalpingography.

Uterus Bicornis with Rudimentary Horn

A rudimentary horn should not be surgically united with its larger
mate, unless the larger one is too small to accommodate a fetus. If the
small horn has no endometrial cavity or if it is not connected with the
cavity of the larger member, there is even less reason for metroplasty.
The entire rudimentary horn should be removed. The weak place left
in the myometrium of the remaining horn must be strengthened and the
remnant of endometrium communicating with the larger cavity must be
found and excised. Reimplantation of the fallopian tube into the other
horn is not recommended. That operation has little chance of success
and may weaken the wall of the remaining horn.

Septate Uterus

Removal of the uterine septum with no other surgical manipulation is
the aim in correcting this malformation. The operation first used by
Ruge in 1884 and recommended by Luikart [10] answers the purpose. Of
vital importance is the determination, in advance of the operation, that
the body of the uterus is not divided. If the uterus is bicornuate and the
operation is carried out (incision of the septum per vaginam), the endometrial cavity will be opened into the peritoneal cavity. In effect the
first step of the Strassman metroplasty will have been accomplished. The
condition of the fundus of the uterus may be determined by visualization
at laparotomy or by culdoscopy.

Luikart surmised that the septum is probably more fibrous than
smooth muscular, and thus less likely to be well supplied with vasculature. On embryologic grounds as well the septum can be expected to
be exactly like the other parts of the myometrium, i.e., smooth muscular.

Surgical Operations for Unification

The aims of surgical correction of the bicornuate uterus are the removal of the partition and the establishment of the uterocervical passageway. There are three different procedures for accomplishing these purposes, the choice of procedure depending upon the configuration of the
uterus to be repaired.

When there are two separate horns converging at about the level of
the internal cervical os, the Strassman metroplasty is best. [14] Using the

abdominal approach, the uterus is incised across its fundal region from a point near one uterotubal junction to a point near the other. The incision enters the endometrial cavities all the way across the "saddle" of the fundus. Traction sutures are placed at the midpoint of the incision, tension on these sutures making the midpoints into ends and the former ends into new midportions. Thus the closure of the myometrium is accomplished with the suture line in the sagittal plane, or at right angle to the direction in which it was made. The shape of the unified uterus is somewhat different from that of a normal uterus in that it is larger in the anteroposterior diameter than in the transverse diameter.

When the uterus is septate or when the body of the uterus is not actually two-horned, the Strassman metroplasty is modified slightly. The incision is made across the fundus of the uterus and carried into both endometrial cavities. The septum is divided with scissors by placing a blade in each cavity and trimming where necessary to remove the ridge of muscular tissue. The incision is repaired in the sagittal direction, preserving all the myometrium and producing the longer ovoid in the anteroposterior direction as well as separating raw surfaces inside the uterus.

When the septate uterus is large enough to allow sacrificing a portion of the myometrium, the procedure recommended by Jones and Jones is useful.[9] These authors prefer to make the initial incision in the sagittal plane, i.e., from front to back of the uterus, excising a thin sliver of myometrium along with the septum. The incision is closed in the same direction in which it was made. Operative trauma does not involve the regions of the uterotubal junctions.

Since operations upon the uterus may be accompanied by considerable bleeding it is useful to place a temporary constriction about the uterine vessels using a small rubber catheter passing through the lower broad ligaments near the level of the cervical junction or lower segment. It is removed at the close of the procedure.

ANOMALOUS MESONEPHRIC STRUCTURES OF THE CERVIX

After its initial contact with the urogenital sinus, the mesonephric duct begins to atrophy in the female fetus of 65-mm, 12-week stage. By the time the fetus has reached a length of 100 mm, the mesonephric ducts are no longer identifiable. In the male fetus, however, the ducts form an ampullary enlargement near their junction with the urogenital sinus. In some females fragmentary remnants may be noted in the region beside the uterovaginal (müllerian) canal. In most adult females the ducts are entirely gone, but in a small number remnants are present in the lateral walls of the cervix.

Ductal remnants may produce small cystic structures which are visible and palpable in or near the vaginal fornices from which they may be excised surgically. However, nearly all instances encountered by us were chance microscopic findings in cervices examined for other conditions, notably specimens removed by sharp conization for early cervical cancer or hysterectomy specimens.

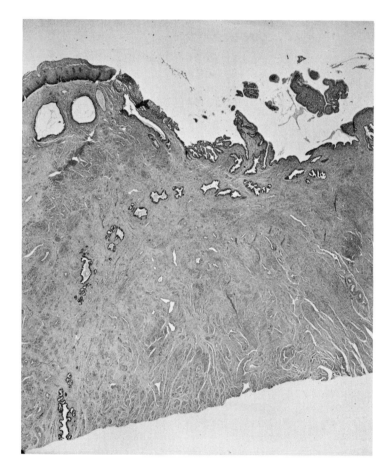

Fig. 8-6. Mesonephric adenosis. Clusters of glandular and tubal epithelium, distinctly different from endocervix, trace curving path through connective tissue body of cervix. Although often found in midlateral zone, mesonephric structures in this specimen approach closely to endocervix. 7×. (From Dougherty, C. M. *Surgical Pathology of Gynecologic Disease*. New York, Harper & Row, 1968.)

In tissue sections the ductal derivatives are often much more proliferated than one might expect of residuals of a simple duct. Indeed, some of the sections show a main channel with many tubular and glandular epithelial passages branching off in all directions. At least two of our specimens (LG62-220 and LG64-15; Figs. 8-6 and 8-7) showed a degree of proliferation and organization which warranted the designation of ampulla (of the vas deferens). In each case the medullary portion of the gonad doubtless produced enough male organizing substance to induce this tiny degree of hermaphroditism—an ampulla of the vas deferens in the female—probably the slightest degree and least productive of symptoms of all varieties of intersexuality.

The course of the residual duct may be straight and parallel to the endocervical canal, at some distance lateral to the endocervix, or it may make a curving approach to the endocervix and reach almost to the mucosa before arching away into the portio vaginalis. In two specimens of cervix examined by us, the duct appeared actually to join the endocervical canal. It would be embryologically disturbing, however, to think that the mesonephric duct ever connected with the müllerian duct!

The epithelium of the ductal remnants is of a small-cell, low columnar type, neatly and evenly arranged. Most of the small spaces on tissue sections are circular in shape, while a few are tubular.

Both adenomatous hyperplasia and adenocarcinoma of mesonephric ductal remnants have been identified in the cervix.[5] The morphologic features of both these proliferative lesions are distinctive. Too few case histories are recorded to allow description of the peculiarities of mesonephric adenocarcinoma.

REFERENCES

1. BAINBRIDGE, W. S. Duplex uterus with multiple pregnancy. *Am J Obstet Gynecol 7*:285, 1924.
2. BRAZE, A. Bicornuate uterus with pregnancy in each horn. *JAMA 123*:474, 1943.
3. CARPENTER, P. J., and POTTER, E. Nuclear sex and genital malformation in 48 cases of renal agenesis, with especial reference to nonspecific female pseudohermaphroditism. *Am J Obstet Gynecol 78*:235, 1959.
4. DORSETT, E. L. Discussion of Luikart. *Am J Obstet Gynecol 31*:797, 1936.
5. DOUGHERTY, C. M. *Surgical Pathology of Gynecologic Disease.* New York, Harper & Row, 1968.
6. FINDLEY, P. Pregnancy in uterus didelphys. *Am J Obstet Gynecol 12*:318, 1926.
7. HINMAN, F., JR. Congenital bilateral absence of the kidneys: Critical review with the report of one additional case. *Surg Gynecol Obstet 71*:101, 1940.

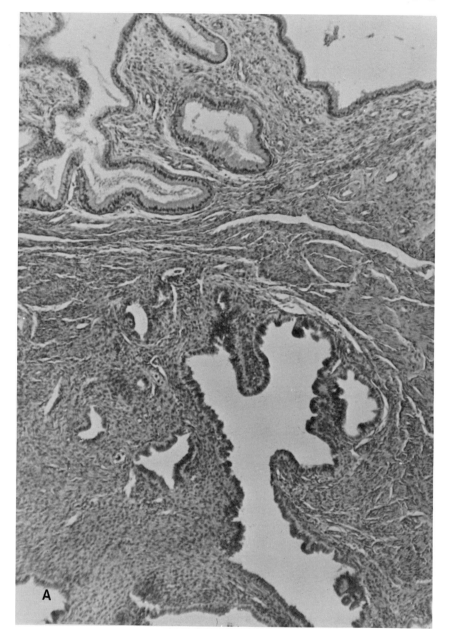

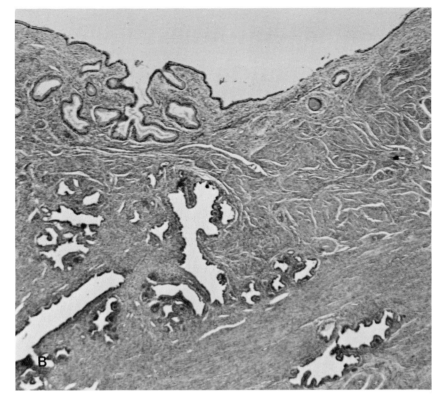

Fig. 8-7. Mesonephric adenosis. *A*. Irregular spaces and clusters of gland-like structures are located deep within connective tissue body of cervix. 24×. *B*. Both types of gland epithelium are seen. Abnormal proliferation of mesonephric elements reaches nearer surface here than usual. 70×. (Parts *A* and *B* from Dougherty, C. M. *Surgical Pathology of Gynecologic Disease*. New York, Harper & Row, 1968.)

8. JARCHO, J. Malformations of the uterus: Review of the subject, including embryology, comparative anatomy, diagnosis and report of cases. *Am J Surg 71*:106, 1946.
9. JONES, H. W., JR., and JONES, G. E. S. Double uterus as an etiological factor in repeated abortion: Indications for surgical repair. *Am J Obstet Gynecol 65*:326, 1953.
10. LUIKART, R. Technic of successful removal of septum of uterus septus and subsequent deliveries at term. *Am J Obstet Gynecol 31*:797, 1936.
11. McKELVEY, J. L., and BAXTER, J. S. Abnormal development of vagina and genitourinary tract. *Am J Obstet Gynecol 31*:797, 1936.
12. ROLEN, A. C., CHOQUETTE, A. J., and SEMMENS, J. P. Rudimentary uterine horn: Obstetric and gynecologic implications. *Obstet Gynecol 27*:806, 1966.

13. SMITH, F. R. Significance of incomplete fusion of the Müllerian ducts in pregnancy and parturition, with report of 35 cases. *Am J Obstet Gynecol 22*:714, 1931.

14. STRASSMAN, P. Die operative Vereinigung eines doppelton Uterus (Nebst Bemerkungen uber die Korrektur der Sogenannten Verdoppelung des Genitalkanales). *Zentralb Gynaekol 31*:1322, 1907.

15. VARINO, G. A., and BEACHAM, W. D. Left renal agenesis, true unicornuate uterus, and total absence of left broad ligament, round ligament, salpinx and ovary. *Am J Obstet Gynecol 41*:124, 1941.

Chapter Nine

Anomalies
of the Vagina

Cary M. Dougherty

Development of the vagina is conditioned by and dependent upon the junction of the müllerian ducts with the urogenital sinus. The point of contact forms the müllerian tubercle. The sinus epithelium appears to be stimulated to proliferate both within the lumen (sinus proliferation) and outside of it (dorsolateral proliferations) at the zone of contact with the blunt müllerian ducts. In the normal process the dorsolateral proliferations of the sinus join in making the midline vaginal cord, a ribbon of epithelium gradually replacing that of the caudal part of the müllerian uterovaginal canal and constituting the framework of the future single vagina. Accordingly, a normal vagina may be expected to indicate a normal cervix and uterus; a double vagina, a double uterus; and absence of the vagina, absence of the uterus.

There are exceptions to this rule, however. For example, the vagina may be partially formed when there is no uterus or cervix, or the uterus may be present with vaginal agenesis. It is, perhaps, unfortunate that the vagina is so readily available to examination, while the remainder of the genital tract is concealed, because the examiner often investigates no further when he finds an anomalous vagina. On the contrary, this discovery mandates a complete diagnostic survey of the genital system and the urorenal apparatus, as well as accurate chromosomal studies. To embark upon a program of surgical operations before accomplishing

TABLE 9-1

CONGENITAL ANOMALIES OF THE VAGINA

Agenesis		11
Absent	8	
Rudimentary	3	
Transverse septum		15
Longitudinal septum (double vagina)		32
Imperforate hymen		11
Anomalous opening of ureter		1
Mesonephric remnants		15 *
Paramesonephric adenosis		1

* Estimated.

thorough diagnostic investigation is to invite unsatisfactory results. Table 9-1 lists the congenital anomalies of the vagina, as the principal organ involved, in the patients in this study. It should be understood that diagnostic studies on most of the patients were incomplete for one reason or another.

AGENESIS OF THE VAGINA

The *absence* of the vagina is usually discovered by the gynecologist when the maturing girl consults him about her failure to start menstruating. Unlike the female who has monthly discomfort and lower abdominal mass due to trapping of menstrual fluid by imperforate hymen or complete transverse septum, the girl who has no vagina usually has no periodic cramps.

Clinical Features

Examination discloses normal or somewhat puerile secondary sex characteristics of adolescence. The mons veneris, pubic hair, and large and small labia are normal. Often there is an actual vestibule recognizable by its pink, moist mucosal lining. The external urethral meatus is located at the usual distance below the clitoris, though it tends to assume a position more or less central to the entire structure of the vulva. Perineum and supporting rectovaginal tissues are present, but there is less space between urethra and anus than when the normal vagina is present.

Hymen

The hymen, as it normally appears at the vaginal introitus, is absent when there is no vagina. This is important, for it seems almost to be the rule that absence of the vagina is first mistakenly diagnosed as imperforate hymen. There may be a somewhat anomalous vaginal vestibule and urethral meatus, but these structures are not derivatives of the vagina and hence are only indirectly affected by vaginal agenesis. When the labia are held apart there is only a sagittal crease in place of the vagina. If the vagina is fully formed with its opening occluded by the intact hymenal membrane, there can be seen a definite rounded, bulging mass within the confines of the labia. Digital rectal examination adds clarifying information in distinguishing agenesis from occlusion of the vagina.

Perineal Body

A transverse muscular support of the perineum is readily identified, though not so deep in the sagittal plane as in the normal case. The *rectovesical space* can be demonstrated by blunt dissection between the two organs. It is composed of loose connective tissue receiving blood supply from small terminal vessels. At the inner boundary of the space, the peritoneum of the pouch of Douglas can be found. If this barrier is torn or incised, the dissected space opens directly into the peritoneal cavity.

Uterus and Tubes

In all except one (CH65-115464) of our patients with agenesis of the vagina in whom inspection of the internal pelvic organs was done, the uterus was absent, vestigial, or rudimentary. In the one exceptional case the patient had a functional uterus even though she also had agenesis of the vagina. A similar case, managed by Dr. L. C. Powell, Jr., Galveston, Texas (Sealy Hospital 134112M), is reported later in this chapter. This combination of anatomic defects leads to medical complications with the onset of menstruation.

Fallopian tubes may be well formed, but are more likely to be of the infantile type, although patent and potentially functional.

Ovaries

Females with vaginal agenesis may or may not possess normal ovaries. As mentioned earlier, failure of development of the vagina may be only part of a more extensive failure of development of genital and urinary systems. While vaginal agenesis does not usually accompany ovarian agenesis, it may do so.

The ovaries may be normally formed to all outward appearances. Incomplete diagnostic studies, however, both in our patients and in those of others, leave doubt about the association of upper and lower genital tract anomalies.

Urorenal System

Of 7 patients with agenesis of the vagina studied by intravenous pyelography, 6 had urinary tract anomalies: 2 had renal agenesis on the right side, 3 had pelvic ectopic kidneys, and 1 had an anomalous kidney pelvis. Other anomalies sometimes found are crossed ectopia and duplication of parts of ureters and kidneys.

Pathogenesis

While not constant, the association of uterocervical agenesis with vaginal agenesis is common enough to indicate that the müllerian ducts must play an inductive role in the sinus proliferation which ultimately forms the vagina. Occasionally the müllerian structures are present but the vagina is absent or the vagina is present but no evidence of müllerian structures can be found. A variation of this same combination of circumstances is seen in the male when the prostatic utricle, a product of the urogenital sinus analogous to the vagina, forms and persists after atrophy of the müllerian ducts.[8,17] In any case, the embryonic structure constituting the beginning of the vagina is a mass of epithelial cells derived from the sinus and forming a solid ribbon of some length between the sinus and the caudal ends of the müllerian ducts. Two possible mechanisms may result in failure of formation of the vagina: (1) the epithelial mass may appear and grow to a certain stage of development, then undergo atrophy and disappear, and (2) the sinus proliferation may not take place as scheduled and hence never form the anlage of the vagina. Both these mechanisms are embryologically possible, and in all probability both occur. If the failure of formation of the vagina were the result simply of failure of canalization of the epithelial mass, abundant epithelial tissue would be found at surgical operation along with cystic remnants and cleavage planes within the tissues which could be recognized by the surgeon. Since such epithelial tissue, abundant or scant, has not been found by operators who have reported their experience,[2] failure of canalization is probably not a mechanism of vaginal agenesis.

The hymen is a crescentic fold of the dorsal wall of the urogenital sinus developed when the greatly enlarging epithelial mass forming the vagina elongates and pushes caudally. When there is no vaginal mass, there is no pressure exerted on the sinus wall and no hymen formed.

The Bartholin glands are not products of the developing vagina but are formed as outgrowths of the urogenital sinus, pars phallica. They may be identified in the area of the vaginal vestibule. Illustrating this point one of our case histories (CH41-17436) described the occurrence of an abscess of the Bartholin gland in a young girl with vaginal agenesis.

Differentiation from Conditions Causing Persistent Urogenital Sinus

Vaginal agenesis may be thought of as causing a state of the lower genitourinary tract like that of persistence of the common urogenital sinus. One of the first investigations must be endoscopic examination of the structure identified as urethra to ascertain whether there is a rudimentary vagina part way up from the external opening. If such a structure is found, the lower "urethra" is, instead, the pars phallica of the urogenital sinus. Helpful aids include urethrography and cystography. Correct identification of the anomaly depends upon evaluation of physical findings in terms of the embryology of the region.

Persistence of the urogenital sinus beyond the 180-mm stage of fetal life is anomalous. In certain babies and girls with masculinization of the genitalia, both vagina and urethra open into a common passageway to the outside. The urethra may be described as opening into the anterior (ventral) vaginal wall, or the vagina may be described as opening into the posterior (dorsal) wall of the urethra, depending upon the relative sizes of the two organs. Both these descriptions are slightly erroneous, however. The meatus of the urethra and the orifice of the vagina are formed at the same level of the urogenital sinus. It would be more correct to consider that they open by a common channel rather than that either opens into the other.

Treatment

Few structures of the human body can be duplicated anatomically as successfully as the vagina. The probable success of the surgical operation, ironically, may be responsible for its hasty performance, in some instances before thorough diagnostic study is completed.

Historically, methods and materials used in reconstruction have included double and single loops of ileum, segments of rectum, pedicle and free skin grafts, and indentation by pressure of graded sizes of glass test tubes.[1, 5, 6, 11] All these procedures have been attended by more or less serious drawbacks. Experience has shown that best results are obtained by blunt dissection of the space between the urethra and bladder and the rectum and anus, followed by primary grafting with a split-thickness graft. A plastic or wood mold of appropriate size is used to hold the graft in place.[10]

Certain technical factors must be considered. The graft must be taken from as hairless an area as can be found, otherwise the new lining may produce hair in its new location as it did originally. Hemostasis must be complete or the graft will not take in the places disrupted by blood clots. Sepsis must be controlled by thorough cleansing of the area and by antibiotic treatment if needed. Scar tissue must be kept at a minimum to prevent contracture of the new vagina. The three most important means of controlling scar formation are those just enumerated: hemostasis, asepsis, and primary grafting.

Finally, the success of the operative reconstruction depends upon the mental preparation and guidance of the patient before and afterward. It would probably be a mistake to construct a vagina in a very young child, as daily care of the artificial organ would not be continued by either child or parent, and contracture would result. Neither should construction be delayed until a prospective male sex partner is at hand. A young woman, told of her anomaly, might prefer to forego marriage entirely so that construction of an artificial vagina would be unnecessary. The gynecologist should consider carefully all the elements in each case before deciding when or whether to perform the surgical operation.

Laparotomy and careful study of the internal genital organs are necessary parts of the treatment of the patient with agenesis of the vagina. If there is a vestigial uterus, it should be removed because there may be vestiges of endometrium also. If, finding a uterus present, the surgeon elects to leave it in situ, he must be careful to see that it is connected to the new vagina.

Hormonal substitution treatment with estrogen is indicated in those patients whose ovaries are not fully functional.

Partial Agenesis

Incomplete development of the vagina results in either a shortened blind pouch extending from the vestibule inward or a short closed segment attached to the portio of the cervix. When the partial vagina consists of the caudal segment only, the diagnostic and therapeutic considerations are similar to those of absence of the vagina. In the typical case the uterus is absent also. Proof of incomplete development of the vagina consists of failure to identify the portio vaginalis of the cervix after competent examination. In the young child or in the individual with infantile genitalia water cystoscopy with an instrument having a Foroblique lens is a satisfactory method of examination.

Treatment of the female with an incomplete vagina depends upon whether and what types of other anomalies are associated. Factors to be considered are generally like those discussed in the case of absence of the vagina.

Agenesis of vagina with uterus present. L65-115464. This 16-year-old
   Negro sought medical help because she had not started menstruating.
   Since the age of 13 years she had had periodic pain about 2 days each

month. She noted growth of pubic and axillary hair for several years, along with moderate breast development. Examination showed her to be a small but apparently normally developing adolescent girl with corresponding secondary sex characteristics. The normally formed external genitalia partially concealed the fact that the vagina was represented by only a dimple between the labia. There were a few stigmata of mongolism, but these were not conclusive for the diagnosis. Pyelography showed incomplete rotation of the right kidney with anomalous formation of the kidney pelvis. Exploratory laparotomy for inspection of the internal genital organs showed them to be essentially normal and functional. The ovaries contained a few cysts and a corpus luteum. Filmy adhesions covering the ovaries and tubes indicated that there probably had been discharge of menstrual fluid through the tubes. No evidence could be seen of hematometra or of encysted blood near the cervix. The surgeon noted no sign of endometriosis.

The patient was scheduled to have vaginoplasty as soon as her mental status was evaluated.

Agenesis of vagina and hematometra in large horn of bicornuate uterus with rudimentary horn. Sealy Hospital No. 134112M. (Patient of Dr. L. C. Powell, Jr., Galveston, Tex.) This 11-year-old Negro consulted the gynecologist because of lower abdominal pain and mass, and failure to menstruate. When examination under anesthesia disclosed absence of the vagina, laparotomy was performed. The uterine fundus was notched, indicating a septum within the endometrial cavity. The right fallopian tube was dilated with old blood. The left kidney possessed fetal lobulations.

The laparotomy was completed by carrying out metroplasty on the bicornuate uterus and tuboplasty on the fimbriated end of the right tube. The left uterine horn was rudimentary and its endometrium vestigial (Fig. 9-1).

The surgical operation was continued by the perineal route where incision of the vaginal vestibule and dissection of the vesicorectal space was done. The cervix was palpated and identified with difficulty, but a continuous canal was established for egress of menstrual blood. Split-thickness skin grafting of the vagina concluded the surgical procedure.

The operator concluded that although there was a well-formed corpus and cervix uteri present with endometrial cavity and cervical canal in the major horn, there was no remnant of the cranial end of the vaginal epithelium. This accounted for the considerable difficulty

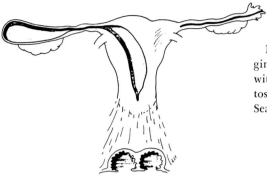

Fig. 9-1. Diagram showing vaginal agenesis, bicornuate uterus with rudimentary horn, hematosalpinx, and hematometra. Sealy Hospital No. 134112 M.

encountered in reaching the endocervix from the perineal surgical approach.

Vaginal agenesis with uterus absent. CH49-350774. A 17-year-old Negro sought medical consultation because she had never menstruated. She reported no significant periodic pains. Examination showed her to be of normal stature for her age, with slightly underdeveloped feminine characteristics. The external genitalia were described as normal for an adolescent girl, except that in place of vaginal opening there was only a slight indentation of tissues. No hymen was present.

Pyelography demonstrated a slightly enlarged left kidney. The right kidney was not visualized. Cystoscopy revealed absence of right ureteral orifice. When examination under anesthesia was done, the examiner did not palpate uterus or ovaries.

The vagina was surgically constructed by dissection of the rectovaginal space and immediate skin grafting using a wooden mold to hold the graft in place. When the mold was removed in 10 days 95 per cent of the graft had taken. Since the donor site of the graft was anterior thigh the vaginal lining was black.

Five months after surgical operation the patient was examined. The vaginal mucosa was healthy and pliable. Scar tissue was minimal. Vaginal cytologic smear showed normal cornification. Pigmentation of the lining was unchanged from its original black color.

Serious complication of skin graft of constructed vagina. CH50-409543. A 17-year-old Caucasian was examined because she had not yet menstruated. The vagina was absent. X-ray showed that the right kidney also was absent, and the left kidney was ectopically located in the pelvis. Laparotomy disclosed that the uterus was absent; the fallopian tubes and ovaries appeared essentially normal. The tubes ended in a fibrous cord near the midline.

An artificial vagina was constructed by dissecting the rectovesical space and applying a skin graft from a medial aspect of the thigh; the graft was held in place by a mold.

Eight years later the patient was reexamined for postcoital spotting. Biopsy of a granular lesion of the vagina showed it to be squamous cell carcinoma. Radiation with radium was carried out but the disease progressed and the patient died of metastasis less than 1 year following diagnosis of carcinoma.

TRANSVERSE SEPTUM OF THE VAGINA

Definition

Sometimes the vagina with a normally formed external aspect may be occluded or partially occluded by a fibroepithelial partition at right angle to the canal and situated at any point along its extent. We reviewed records of 15 patients who had transverse septa of the vagina as the main developmental anomaly of the genital tract.

Types of Transverse Septa

In most patients the septum appears as a thin diaphragm-like structure which seems to cause the vagina to end blindly. Close examination may show a small opening or hole in the septum through which fluid is permitted to drain. The hole may be described as "pin-point," or "the size of a pencil," or it may admit a small probe. The anomaly sometimes takes the form of a constriction or stenosis of the vagina by a thick fibrous band which is resistant to stretching. Sometimes the vagina does, indeed, end blindly against a thick mass of tissue which completely blocks the canal and prevents drainage.

Associated Developmental Defects

As noted earlier, agenesis of the vagina and double vagina are associated with faults of other parts of the genital tract. Not so with transverse septum of the vagina. In all our patients in whom information was available the internal genital organs were normal, and in a number of cases pregnancy occurred.

Pathogenesis

There are two embryologic explanations for the formation of a transverse vaginal septum. In the formation of the vagina the müllerian ducts grow caudally until they abut the urogenital sinus, where they indent the wall and apparently stimulate proliferation of the sinus epithelium. The sinus epithelium proliferates into a tongue of tissue extending along the same pathway which was used by the müllerian ducts in moving caudally, only now the movement is back toward the head with the sinus epithelium pushing against the müllerian epithelium if not actually displacing it. When the tract of new epithelial growth is fully developed, it begins to acquire a central lumen from caudal to cranial direction. One explanation for transverse vaginal septum is imperfect displacement of the müllerian epithelium with consequent stricture production at the point of contact of the two epithelial masses. This explanation is plausible on the basis of the older concept that the vagina is in a large part müllerian,[9] but the second explanation, failure of complete canalization of the epithelial mass of the vagina, is both simpler and more in keeping with newer ideas of the embryology of the vagina.

Very likely, both mechanisms occur. Even though the vagina is now believed to be totally of sinus origin in the normal fetus, the process of sinus proliferation and vaginal plate formation might be interfered with or arrested before it accomplishes complete replacement of müllerian epithelium with that of sinus derivation. In such a case there may be a sinus-müllerian junction somewhere along the vaginal tract with stricture or septum formation.

Clinical Features

This condition is nearly always discovered in the young girl in her late teens or early twenties. Since the external genitalia, including the vaginal orifice are normal, there is no reason to suspect the presence of the septum until it interferes either with menstruation or with coitus. If the septum does not block egress of menstrual fluid and if it is not an obstacle to coitus it may not be detected until the time of a routine examination. In a number of our patients the condition was first found at an initial prepartum check-up. Study of our case histories suggest that it is the vaginal band rather than the septum which is discovered at the routine examination.

The location of the septum follows no rule. It may be situated at any point along the vaginal canal, from cervix to introitus. In most of our patients the septum was in the lower third of the canal, although other observers have found more situated in the upper third.[7]

It is often the case that the transverse septum does not completely partition the vagina. Only a portion of the patients give a history of amenorrhea. Those who do have obstruction have the same symptoms as the patient with imperforate hymen or with normal uterus and vaginal agenesis. There is periodic monthly pain in the lower abdomen lasting for a few days, and sometimes the gradual formation of a mass palpable abdominally and rectally. Three of our patients developed hematometrocolpos. If suppuration-causing microorganisms gain entrance to the encysted bloody fluid, a pelvic abscess results, as in one of our patients.

The diagnostic work-up of the patient must differentiate vaginal septum from partial agenesis. In agenesis the vagina may end in a short blind pouch, and usually the uterus is either rudimentary or absent. In the case of vaginal septum an upper segment of vagina communicates with an intact cervix and uterus.

Complications of vaginal septum, in addition to entrapping of menstrual fluid, may be infertility or dystocia. Two of our patients were delivered by cesarean section when the obstetrician thought vaginal delivery not feasible. The problem of dystocia was studied by Burkhart,[3] who concluded that although difficulty in vaginal delivery may be encountered in the occasional case, pregnancy seemed to cause softening of the stenotic band and thus prepared the way for the vaginal delivery.

Treatment

When the condition is stenosis caused by a fibromuscular band of the vaginal wall treatment may be unnecessary, as coitus may produce enough dilation. If the band is too rigid it may be incised in three or four places with short longitudinal incisions which are closed transversely. Excision of the band with an annular segment of vaginal wall has been recommended by TeLinde.[16] It should be noted that this procedure carries the potential hazard of fistula formation and possible failure if a cicatricial band forms in the site of the excision.

The thin fibroepithelial septum may be stretched or lightly torn away. If it is too thick or too vascular for dilation, it may be incised with cross-shaped incisions and hem-stitched with interrupted stitches to prevent stricture.

If the surgical removal of a vaginal septum is done in an unmarried girl, it is important that she return frequently thereafter for digital dilation. It may be advisable to have a plastic mold fitted until healing is complete.

Occasionally a firm or rigid vaginal band in a gravid individual may necessitate cesarean delivery.

Transverse vaginal septum with hematocolpos. CH50-402579. A 12-year-old Negro was seen in the emergency room of the hospital for lower

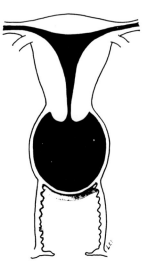

Fig. 9-2. Diagram showing transverse septum of vagina with hematocolpos and hematometra. CH50-
402579.

abdominal pain of 3 days duration. She stated she had never had a
menstrual period. The examining gynecologist found a firm mass
filling the pelvis and extending up into the lower abdominal cavity.
The external genitalia were sexually mature. The hymen was identified and found to be patent. A short distance inside the vagina, the
examiner found a bulging tense cystic mass. With the patient under
general anesthesia a cross-shaped incision was made and about 500 ml
of old menstrual blood drained (Fig. 9-2).

After a 6-weeks' interval the patient was readmitted to the hospital
and the septum was excised. The vaginal mucosa was sutured in the
area of the defect, in the manner of anastamosis of intestine. Healing
was satisfactory without evidence of cicatrix.

Fibroepithelial vaginal septum with small opening causing dyspareunia.
CH65-96474. An 18-year-old Caucasian complained of inability to have
coitus after 4 months of marriage. Menstruation was said to be normal, each period accompanied by moderate cramping. Examination
showed the patient to be normally developed for her age. The external genitalia were of the normal mature type. The vagina was approximately 1 in. deep, but at the apex there was a small opening
through which a sound could be inserted for 4–5 in. more.

Laparotomy for inspection of internal organs showed functional
ovaries, normal tubes, and fully formed uterus with cervix. From the
vaginal approach the apex of the vagina was opened and dissected
for a short distance until it opened onto the portio vaginalis of the

cervix. A large mold was placed in the vagina. The raw areas of the upper vagina were eventually epithelized by upgrowth of vaginal epithelium.

IMPERFORATE HYMEN

Normal Structure

The hymen is developed as a lunate fold produced when the plunger-like mass of vaginal epithelium elongates caudally and presses against the dorsal wall of the urogenital sinus. It is formed from a dorsal ("posterior") segment and two lateral segments. There is no significant hymenal structure attached at the urethral meatus, except when the membrane has no opening—the imperforate hymen. The size of the hymen varies from a vestigial thin veil of tissue left over at the junctional seam of the vestibule (urogenital sinus) and the vaginal tube to a completely intact diaphragm-like membrane. When the hymenal membrane is prominent, the small opening is almost always found just below (dorsal to) the urethra. Thus, the shape of the hymen is still lunate, though the crescent is deeper, with the dorsal or posterior segment making up most of the membrane.

That the hymen is a relatively unimportant vestigial part of the vagina is clear from the ease and painlessness with which it is stretched in two particular instances: The opening is 1.5–2 cm in diameter in adolescent girls who have used vaginal menstrual tampons, and in females who have engaged in coitus the hymenal opening is several centimeters in diameter.

Pathogenesis

The hymen may be imperforate by error of development, or it may undergo conglutination in the same manner as adhesion of the labia minora of the vulva. After the extreme proliferation and growth of the sinus epithelium forms the mass from which the vagina is to be shaped, the vaginal lumen is brought into being by central cavitation of the epithelial mass. If the central cavity stops short of the caudal extent of the vagina, the lumen does not connect with that of the sinus, i.e., the hymen is imperforate. The hymen is usually only a thin membrane when it is imperforate by error of development.

Conglutination of the orifice of the hymen may result from inflammatory reaction or other chronic irritative influences. In this case there is other evidence of damage, as thickening of the labia or adhesions about the clitoris.

Clinical Features

There were 11 case histories on file with sufficient information recorded to substantiate the diagnosis of imperforate hymen. All patients
were in their early teens when seen and treated by the gynecologic
service. The stories in all cases were similar.

The patient consults the gynecologist because of her failure to start
menstruation. She notes periodic lower abdominal pain and development of a mass in the lower abdomen. If the enlarging mass presses on
the urethra, the patient has retention of urine with attendant symptoms.

Examination shows the patient to be a normal adolescent girl with
secondary sex characteristics usual to the age. External genitalia are
well formed. The hymen is represented by a complete diaphragm across
the vaginal opening. The membrane is pink but the collection of old
blood behind it imparts a blue-black tint to the hymen, while the pressure of accumulated fluid produces outward bulging. Rectal-abdominal
palpation confirms the presence of the mass distending the vagina. Under
favorable conditions of examination the gynecologist is able to palpate
the small uterus displaced upward by the mass.

Differentiation from Agenesis of the Vagina

Imperforate hymen and hematocolpos are never mistaken for agenesis
of the vagina, but vaginal agenesis may be mistaken by the inexperienced
physician for imperforate hymen. Imperforate hymen is easily recognized
by the obvious signs: the normally formed external genitalia, the well
developed vaginal vestibule, the recognizable hymen, and the pelvic-
abdominal mass are diagnostic. If there is doubt in the mind of the
examiner the patient must be studied more carefully for other features
of vaginal agenesis. It should be emphasized that of the two conditions,
vaginal agenesis is of far more grave concern to the patient and doctor.

Treatment

The correct treatment is incision or excision of the hymen, with institution of safeguards to prevent closure of the wound. It may be useful
to confirm the diagnosis of encysted menstrual blood by inserting a
large-bore needle through the membrane and aspirating a sample of
the contents. Incision is usually made in the form of a cross with the
limbs extending to the junction of hymen with vaginal wall. If hemo-
static sutures are necessary, interrupted stitches of fine absorbable material should be used rather than a continuous running stitch which
would tend to narrow the opening.

If the surgeon elects to excise all or a portion of the hymenal membrane, a zig-zag or undulating line of excision should be used to prevent

development of an annular scar. A satisfactory partial excision can be carried out from the initial cruciate incision by trimming off parts of the four points created by the incision.

It is important to inspect the hymen periodically during the healing in order to dilate the opening if necessary.

Complications

Complications caused by the accumulation of encysted bloody fluid include pain and swelling, acute urinary retention, and damage to the epithelial linings of the vagina, cervix, and uterus. These linings may be partially replaced by granulation-type tissue in a natural response to the attempted removal of the blood.

Complications after treatment include recurrence of atresia and hematocolpos, annular scar formation, and dyspareunia.

Associated Anomalies

Other developmental defects are not associated with imperforate hymen as they are with vaginal agenesis. Although work-up was not complete in all our patients, some later proved the capability of their organs by having children, four born to two mothers at last count.

Imperforate hymen: Initial surgical incision closed, hematocolpos recurred. CH51-24925. A 13-year-old Negro, born at Charity Hospital, suffered cramping in the lower abdomen. She was normally developed for an adolescent. Examination disclosed a bulging hymen. The hymen was incised, clots and dark blood were removed from the vagina, and the patient was sent home after a week's hospitalization (Fig. 9-3).

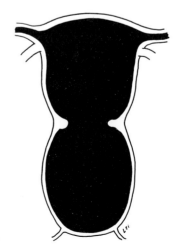

Fig. 9-3. Diagrammatic representation of imperforate hymen with hematocolpos and hematometra. CH51-24925.

Two months later symptoms recurred. Examination showed that the opening in the hymen had sealed again and the hematocolpos had recurred. The surgeon removed most of the hymen this time, and the patient, followed carefully for over a year, remained well.

Imperforate hymen with urinary retention as admitting symptom. CH44-133363. This 12-year-old Negro came in to the hospital because she was unable to urinate. Examination showed normal beginning sexual maturation and well-developed and maturing external genitalia. The labia minora were held apart slightly by a prominent bulging hymen, which appeared to the examiner as if it concealed an accumulation of old blood within. The hymen was excised and the mucosa sutured. Examination disclosed the vagina and cervix to be greatly dilated, the corpus uteri about normal size. The patient had at least three successful pregnancies after hymenectomy.

ANOMALOUS GLAND STRUCTURES OF THE VAGINA

Mesonephric Ductal Derivatives

The mesonephric duct reaches its maximum point of development in the female fetus of about 40–45 mm, its lumen continuous with the lumen of the urogenital sinus. In the pelvic region the paired ducts are immediately lateral to the caudal end of the fused müllerian ducts. When the sinus epithelium begins to proliferate to form the vaginal cord or plate, the wolffian ducts slowly regress. In the 65-mm fetus the mesonephric ducts are well on their way to atrophy as the vaginal cell mass elongates. In the usual situation the mesonephric ducts which occupy a position beside the vaginal cord disappear completely with no remnant visible by about the 100-mm stage. In the exceptional case, however, the mesonephric duct may persist in this location and in later life form a vestigial tract from vaginal fornix to hymenal ring. This fetal residual has been referred to as Gartner's duct in the adult female.

In the mature female the usual evidence of residual vestige of the mesonephric duct is the solitary cyst protruding into the vaginal lumen. The cysts are most often solitary and occupy a posterolateral position in relation to the vagina. Occasionally two or more cysts may be seen in the same individual.

The microscopic structure of the lining of the mesonephric cyst is not distinctive and may be somewhat variable. The typical mesonephric-type epithelium is composed of low columnar cells of nonsecretory type.

It may be that the variability of form of this epithelium as described by medical writers is due to the fact that most vaginal cysts are called cysts of Gartner's duct whether they arise in mesonephric ductal remnants or other glandular structures.

Mesonephric adenocarcinoma has been identified in the vagina, the identification being largely on histologic characteristics.[12, 13]

Müllerian Ductal Derivatives

Mucous columnar epithelium typical of the endocervix has been found growing within the vaginal wall beneath the mucosa or actually on the surface of the vagina in a manner similar to its occurrence in the endocervix. Two mechanisms may account for this dislocation of tissues, one congenital and one acquired.

In the early development of the vagina the two müllerian ducts first join in the midline and extend all the way caudally to the wall of the urogenital sinus. There a sustained proliferation of the sinus epithelium causes the müllerian epithelium to recede, or appear to recede, as its place is taken by the sinus upgrowth. The junction of the müllerian epithelium and sinus epithelium is, to say the least, labiie, and portions of müllerian epithelium might easily come to occupy sites within the vaginal anlage. In later life the displaced epithelium may undergo proliferation and mucification.

The acquired mechanism involves growth of the endocervical epithelium out onto the upper vagina in the same way it spreads onto the portio vaginalis of the cervix. This mechanism explains the location of endocervical epithelium on the surface of the vagina, though it does not so readily account for the gland spaces within the vaginal wall.

The term paramesonephric adenosis of the vagina has been used to designate the condition of surface as well as submerged glandular epithelium of müllerian type.[4] When there is extensive replacement of stratified squamous epithelium by mucinous epithelium in the vagina, there is excessive vaginal discharge of mucus, but no other distinguishing signs (Fig. 9-4). Closed spaces within the vaginal wall lined by mucus-secreting epithelium result in cyst formation. Studdiford reported multiple small shot-like nodules found on the posterior vaginal wall, some of which were visible through the mucosa as vesicles.[15]

Solitary cysts of the vagina are more often of the mucinous epithelial type. They are rarely more than moderate in size, and are removed surgically without difficulty, either by excision or marsupialization.

Malignant change in the glandular structures in the vagina is rare, but adenocarcinoma of müllerian type histologically has been reported.

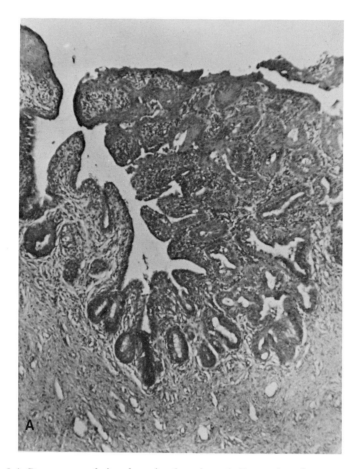

Fig. 9-4. Paramesonephric adenosis of vagina. *A.* Parts of surface present pattern of clefts and folds seen in endocervix, with intermingling of the two types of cervical epithelium. 70×. *B.* Relation of squamous epithelium to mucous columnar lining of glands is same as that in cervix in erosion healing. Strip of basal epithelial cells may be seen under columnar lining of a gland space. 70×. (Parts *A* and *B* from Dougherty, C. M. *Surgical Pathology of Gynecologic Disease.* New York, Harper & Row, 1968.)

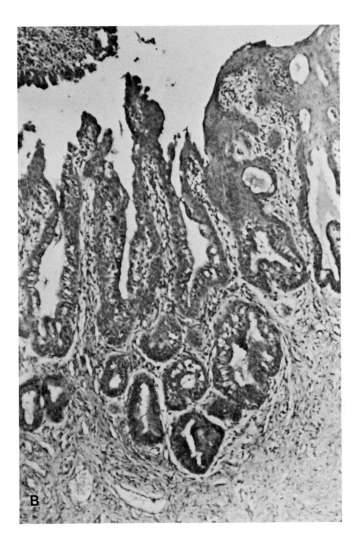

TABLE 9-2

OCCURRENCE OF DOUBLE VAGINA IN ASSOCIATION WITH VARIOUS
UTERINE MALFORMATIONS AND WITH NORMAL UTERUS

Type of Uterus	Total No. of Patients	No. with Double Vagina
Didelphys	22	20
Bicornis unicollis	30	3
Bicornis (unspecified)	19	1
Normal		8 *

* In three patients, one of the double vaginas ended blindly; in two the septum was incomplete.

LONGITUDINAL SEPTUM OF THE VAGINA (DOUBLE VAGINA)

The vagina may be divided by a sagittal partition into approximately equal or into unequal compartments. The partition may extend the length of the vagina from hymen to portio vaginalis of the cervix, or it may be incomplete in its upper or its lower extent. Potter [14] mentioned a longitudinal septum attached from side to side of the vagina, separating it into ventral and dorsal compartments. This condition has not been seen by us. Table 9-2 lists the number of patients with double vagina studied by us.

Double vagina is usually found in association with uterus didelphys (Fig. 8-1). The vaginal septum begins at the hymen, dividing it into two halves, and is continuous with the partition in the cervix and uterus. As shown in Table 9-2, however, there are a number of variations.

Pathogenesis

Two factors in development of the genital tract make it possible for the vagina to be formed with a partition: (1) the pelvic portions of the paired müllerian ducts normally fuse into a single channel, the primitive genital canal or the uterovaginal canal; and (2) the vagina is first formed from paired sinus epithelial proliferations separated by a thin sliver of mesenchyme. The usual process of coalescence brings both the ducts and the proliferations into single structures; failure of coalescence allows the persistence of the more primitive bipartite state.

The extent to which the müllerian ducts condition the subsequent development of the vagina is clear from the usual association of single uterus with single vagina and double uterus with double vagina. The exceptional occurrence must be noted, however, of vagina with no uterus, single vagina with double uterus, and double vagina with single uterus.

Clinical Features

There may be no symptoms leading the patient to suspect that she has an anomalous lower genital tract. In the exceptional case dyspareunia may raise the suspicion. Dystocia and immediate postpartal bleeding from laceration may signal obstetric complications caused by longitudinal septum. Infertility could result if one compartment of a double vagina ended in a blind pouch and if the sex partner used this noncommunicating sheath.

Treatment

The presence of a longitudinal septum of the vagina does not of itself demand treatment. Excision of the septum should be done when there are symptoms. The septum may be removed by a single incision or by removing a longitudinal strip from its entire length. It is preferable to make the incision under direct vision and to ligate bleeding points, rather than to clamp and ligate in a step by step procedure. Bleeding from vaginal arterial branches may be expected, but the vessels may be clamped as they are severed. After completion of the incision the mucosal edges are approximated with a continuous suture.

If a wide band of tissue is removed the length of the septum, there is the chance that a fistula may form or that the resulting single vagina may be of too small diameter.

REFERENCES

1. BALDWIN, J. F. Formation of an artificial vagina by intestinal transplantation. *Am J Obstet Gynecol 56:*636, 1907.
2. BRYAN, A. L., NIGRO, J. A., and COUNSELLER, V. S. One hundred cases of congenital absence of vagina. *Surg Gynecol Obstet 88:*79, 1949.
3. BURKHART, K. P. Vaginal soft-tissue dystocia. *Obstet Gynecol 20:*808, 1962.
4. DOUGHERTY, C. M. Histopathology of surgically excised lesions of the vagina. *Ann NY Acad Sci 83:*328, 1959.
5. FRANK, R. T. The formation of an artificial vagina without operation. *Am J Obstet Gynecol 35:*1053, 1938.
6. GRAD, H. The technique of formation of artificial vagina. *Surg Gynecol Obstet 54:*200, 1932.
7. JONES, H. W., JR., and SCOTT, W. W. *Hermaphroditism, Genital Anomalies and Related Endocrine Disorders.* Baltimore, Williams & Wilkins, 1958, p. 334.
8. JOST, A. Embryonic Sexual Differentiation (Morphology, Physiology, Abnormalities). In Jones, H. W., Jr., and Scott, W. W. *Hermaphroditism, Genital Anomalies and Related Endocrine Disorders.* Baltimore, Williams & Wilkins, 1958, p. 33.

9. KOFF, A. K. Development of the vagina in the human fetus. *Contrib Embryol* 25:59, 1933.

10. MARSHALL, G. B. Artificial vagina: A review of the various operative procedures for correcting atresia vaginae. *J. Obstet Gynaecol Br Emp 23:* 193, 1913.

11. McINDOE, A. H., and BANISTER, J. B. An operation for the cure of congenital absence of the vagina. *J Obstet Gynaecol Br Emp 45:*490, 1938.

12. MEYER, R. Uber adenom- und Karzinombildung an der Ampulla des Gartnerschen Ganges. *Virchows Arch Pathol Anat 174:*270, 1903.

13. NOVAK, E., WOODRUFF, D., and NOVAK, E. Probable mesonephric origin of certain female genital tumors. *Am J Obstet Gynecol 68:*1222, 1954.

14. POTTER, E. L. *Pathology of the Fetus and the Newborn.* Chicago, Year Book, 1952, p. 386.

15. STUDDIFORD, W. E. Vaginal lesions of adenomatous origin. *Am J Obstet Gynecol 73:*641, 1957.

16. TeLINDE, R. In Jones, H. W., Jr., and Scott, W. W., *op. cit.,* p. 337.

17. VILAS, E. Uber die Entwicklung der Uticulus prostaticus beim Menschen, *Z Anat Entwicklungsgesch 99:*599, 1933.

Index

72 73 74 75 76 10 9 8 7 6 5 4 3 2 1